The Secret Journey

Paul Christian

Published by
Melange Books, LLC
White Bear Lake, MN 55110
www.melange-books.com

The Secret Journey, Copyright © 2012 by Paul Christian

Print ISBN: 978-1-61235-353-1

Names, characters, and incidents depicted in this book are products of the author's imagination or are used fictitiously. Any resemblance to actual events, locales, organizations, or persons, living or dead, is entirely coincidental and beyond the intent of the author or the publisher. No part of this book may be reproduced or transmitted in any form or by any means, electronic or mechanical, including photocopying, recording, or by any information storage and retrieval system, without permission in writing from the publisher.
Published in the United States of America.

Cover Art by Caroline Andrus

For Honey

About the author:

Paul Christian is a creation of your imagination. He lives where your desire touches your reality, and he is everything you dream him to be.

www.the-secret-journey.com

The Secret Journey
Paul Christian

"Yeah I want you, spread on my bed like a banquet..."

With these words, author Paul Christian starts weaving a web of seduction that inexorably draws the reader into his dark and intensely erotic world. The line between fantasy and reality blurs, grows faint, and is finally broken as he beguiles the reader into a compelling sexual exploration unlike any other. Half narrative, half love letter, The Secret Journey is not a story but an experience, arousing, hypnotic, and relentlessly compelling. It is a masterwork destined to stand with the classics of erotic literature.

Table of Contents

Ab Initio — 7
The Bath — 13
Part Two — 17
The Trainer — 29
Part Three — 35
The Traveller — 49
Part Four — 55
The Teacher — 63
Part Five — 77
Cage Girl — 81
Part Six — 87
Bike Girl — 111
Part Seven — 117
Bike Girl II — 125
Part Eight — 131
Bike Girl III — 137
Part Nine — 143
Dance Girl — 151
Part Ten — 155
Surf Girl — 167
Part Eleven — 171
The Buyer — 173
Part Twelve — 183
The Writer — 221
Au Revoir — 231

Ab Initio

Yeah I want you. I want you, spread on my bed like a banquet, to feed the hunger of my lust, and quench the thirst of my desire. I want you like nothing else and I'm going to have you too. I'm going to have you right now, just take you, just make you do exactly everything you want so much for me to make you do. What I love is the way your pupils dilate when I say that, when you read that. What I love is the way your breathing quickens ever so slightly, the way your lips part, suddenly dry.

Right now, this time, this place, it's just you and me, alone and private. This is our time and nothing else counts, all the rules are gone. You aren't reading this when and where I'm writing it, but it's still the same thought, the same words surging from my mind and into you, into the fertile womb of your imagination. I don't know you, not even your name. I can't see you, can't hear you, but I can feel you out there and I am going to have you, oh yes, oh yes. I don't give a damn about your husband or your boyfriend or your girlfriend, and I care less what your family and your neighbours and your friends might think. This is about you and me, and nothing matters but the fact that you're a ripe and fertile woman and I'm a man strong enough and smart enough to have you like this. You can deny it if you want and maybe you are, but you've licked your parted lips by now and you're not going to stop reading. You don't want the phone to ring, you don't want a friend to visit. You're mine and I'm already taking you exactly where you need to be taken and you don't want it to stop.

No you don't want it to stop at all, what you want is more, and more, and more. You want to feel my hands in your hair, pulling your head back. You want your lips parted and my mouth on yours to take your gasp away. You want to be plundered like pirate treasure and you know that's just what's going to happen, and you can feel your nipples firming at the thought. And yes, your crotch is getting wet as you feel the desire to slide your hand down to your eager swelling clit. You want that more than anything, and you know how good it's going to feel to slide your finger over it, teasing, teasing, then up inside, up between your moist and pouting folds. But you're not going to, no you're not. You're not going to because I don't want you to and while we do this you're going to do exactly what I want. That's the way it's going to work, that's the game and we're already playing, and you don't have to admit you like it because I already know you do, or you wouldn't still be here now.

Understand, this isn't complicated. No it's very simple, very basic. You'll get no roses in the morning, no shy glances, soft caresses. I don't care what you want, but I know what you need and I know I need to give it to you, oh yes, oh so hard, and oh so deep. And you can deny it if you like but you're wet now and what I want is your hands on your breasts, touching them, stroking them, so warm and alive, soft and feminine. Do it, right now, fingertips grazing that soft, beautiful flesh. Now, right *now*. Don't touch your nipples, though I know they're already ready, eager for the slightest touch. Just feel your tits, so round and firm, and now weigh them, press them, squeeze them. Squeeze them hard, fingers digging in like mine would, like mine will, like I owned them. Don't be gentle, don't even try. Do it hard, very hard, hard enough to make you gasp and then do it harder. You don't want gentle, you want rough and you only wish I'd let you do this to your nipples too, hard now themselves, aching, pointing, eager for their own turn. You only wish I was right there to do it for you, do that and so much more. You want me to just get on with it, take them, tug them, squeeze them till the thrill soaks your cunt, squeeze them till you gasp, squeeze them till they hurt and you want it to stop and I do it harder anyway and your knees go weak and you know you're mine, know it deep in your cunt, your moist and hungry cunt, swelling now, clit firm and ready and getting wetter every second.

Yeah you want that on your nipples, you know it and I know it and I want you to say it, say it right now, say it out loud. "Yes." Go on, say it. Say it because this won't work if you don't and you've gone too far to back out now. Say it because you want to say it, say it because you need it to say it. Don't read another line until you've said it to me, out loud.
"Yes."

Out loud. Taste the word on your tongue.
"Yes."

And I can hear the tremble in your voice, hear the catch in the whisper. Say it again, say it louder this time, like you mean it, like you need it.
"Yes."

And the word releases you. Oh yes, I hear you, honey, and yes I do love to hear you say it, and yes you can, yes you can slide your fingers over your ripe, firm nipples. Feel them anxious, upturned, needy, getting harder beneath your fingertips. Squeeze them gently, feel them stiff and proud, feel your back arch to press your breasts forward into your hands. Squeeze them more, feel the pressure build and build, right up to the edge. Hold them there, lift your breasts with them. You like that, don't you? You like showing off your lovely tits like that, so ripe and full and sensitive. You want more, I know you do, greedy woman that you are. You want it all, you want everything and everything is exactly what you're going to get. Go on, you know how to get more by now, don't you. Say it…

"Yes."

Oh honey, you can do better than that, you can do so much better than that. You don't want it if you can't say it better than that. Go on, try again, louder, clearer.

"Yes."

Like you mean it.

"Yes!"

Like you need it!

"YES!"

And that was better, and yes I do love to hear it, but yes is not enough, not anymore. Let's try…

"Please"

That's what I want from you, what I want to hear from your trembling lips. Lick them for me because they're dry again, and say it for me once again, say it because you want it, say it because you need it, say it because you know how much it turns me on to hear you say it.

"Please."

And now you've said it, think about what you look like - breathing faster, teasing your nipples, squeezing them hard and begging for it harder. How do they feel - hard and swollen and sore and sensitive and aching, aching for more. How do you feel - sexy, slutty, slighty crazy to be doing this, but you're doing it and you're going to keep doing it till I'm done with you. Think about how it makes you feel to say it one more time, how it makes you feel to give yourself like that, begging for it harder on your swollen, aching nipples.

"Please"

Oh that's so beautiful to hear. And think about how it makes me feel to know you're saying it. Think about what it's like for me. Think about how much I love knowing exactly what I'm doing to you, how much I love it that I can have you just like this. Come on, honey, convince me that you want it.

"Please, please, please. Please let me tease them, squeeze them. Please let me please you with them, please, please, *please*."

And since you asked so nicely, yes you can. Pinch them, twist them hard, hard, harder. Twist them till you gasp, and yes I love the sound of that even more than the sound of 'Please', though that's still on your lips now, it won't leave them, "Please please*please*", mixed around the gasps and groans and yes I love the sound of you giving in, giving yourself over to the moment, over to me. Your cunt is soaked now, soaked and still getting wetter and your hips need to move, need to rock. They won't stay still, can't stay still, feel them respond as you respond. And what you want right now, what you crave, what you need, is not seduction, not romance. What you want, what you need, what you crave right now is nothing more or less than for me to fuck you. My hands on your hips, hard on the swell of your ass, spreading you, exposing you, opening you for my cock. And you know what I want to hear as you slide your hand down to your swollen ready clit.

"Fuck me."

Yeah, slide it down there, honey. Slide it up and down and feel the need, feel the thrill. And God, I love it when you say that, demanding, pleading, eager, willing. Let me hear it.

"Fuck me."

And what I love is the glisten of your cunt and the way its scent goes straight to the back of my brain and tells me to hurry up and get inside you, deep, deep in you, claiming you, possessing you, making you mine, all mine. And what I love is the way your legs just open automatically, the way your hips move up to present your perfect pussy - framed by your ass and thighs like living art. And what I love is the need in your voice, the wild, trembling need revealed as you rub your clit in desperation. Say it for me honey.

"Please fuck me. Please"

And there's nothing like the instant when I thrust it in and I don't care if what I hear is pain or pleasure and I doubt you know yourself. I'm not here to treat you gently, I am here to spread you, take you, make you, fill you, use you, stretch you tight around my rigid, thrusting throbbing cock. Feel it, feel it pounding in you, tearing from your throat the words you can't contain.

"Please oh please oh fuck me hard hard *hard*!"

And I am here to slam it in you because you are exactly what I need right now, spread and wet and full and fucked. And I don't care if it hurts you or it hurts me, I'm just here to make you scream and make you beg and I don't care that you'll lose your mind to your bursting clit. I just care that you're right there, right now, your perfect ass at the perfect angle and your perfect cunt rammed full of cock. I am going hold you there and keep you there and fuck you hard and harder still until I'm done, and the only thing that makes it better is to hear your pre-orgasmic cry.

"Fuck me oh my fucking god *please* fuck me fuck me*fuckme*!"

But guess what, honey. It wouldn't matter what you said because the only thing that's going to happen is that I'm going to fuck you just that hard, just pound your cunt until the words are blenderized, until you can't speak, can't see, can't move, can't think. Until the only thing in your entire world is to take it, take it, take it for me, just raise your ass and spread yourself, give me everything, until I give that final rigid thrust into your deepest, secret depths and flood your hungry, fertile cunt, unload my balls into you with such intensity I cannot help but roar. And what I want is your orgasm, clenching hard around my rigid, pumping rod. What I want is to feel you stiffen, see you shake and scream and cry and tear the sheets in ecstasy and see the world go black and fall into delirium knowing that you're mine, mine, *mine*. What I want is your orgasm and I want it right now. Now!

And what I want is to taste your sweat and to see your trembling, sated body lying tangled next to mine. And what I love is the way you breathe and the curve of your breast and the flush of your cheek and your deep, deep eyes. And what I love is the fact that I'm the one who took you there and it matters not the slightest bit that I took you there in text.

And I know you think it's over now, but it isn't, no, it's only just begun. You're like Bambi in the headlights, honey, and you don't even know that it's too late to dodge the truck. You're there alone, there all warm and post orgasmic and it's only innocent masturbation, private sex with just yourself and some book you picked up, and no-one else will ever know. You think that these are only words, but honey, words have power, words change lives. This is about you and me, and my words have just changed your life because from now until forever you have only two choices, and choice one is to put this book down and walk away and never pick it up again, and choice two is to keep turning pages, in the full knowledge that I'm not going to just change your life, I'm going to remake it. I'm going to find out who you are, and I'm going take you where I want to take you and make you complicit in your own seduction. I'm going to do that because I am real, as real as you are. I am right here on the other side of this page, looking out as you look in. Look at the door, wherever you are, look at the door to your room or your office or your car, look at the door, look at it right now and realize that I'm on the other side of it. Through that door is a journey, our journey, and I'm going to take you places you can't yet imagine.

And because you're still here reading I know I've gotten to you. You're fascinated by this little interaction, compelled by it and right now you can't even bother to deny it. This part is *Ab Initio*, - 'From the Beginning', and this is the beginning of the journey, honey, this is the start of the road. The question is, can you handle it? Yes or no, stop or go? It's up to you, honey. Are you up for it? Are you going to turn the page, open the door, take that next step?

We're about to find out.

The Bath

End of the day, sweaty, dirty, tired and stressed, angry at work, angry at the world, in no mood for this, in no mood for anything, sullen, defiant but there - standing in the bathroom, waiting for the bath. Water running, shower spouting pure hot, steaming, spraying, splashing, heating up the tub and tiles and the warm moist air wraps around you like a blanket, bath salts smelling like cinnamon. The tub begins to fill and you hope the water won't be too hot. Turned around to face the other way, hands from behind undo your buttons, pants fall to your ankles, shirt off over your head. No co-operation is necessary, no fussing is allowed. Bra strap popped, breasts come free, one foot lifted out of your puddled clothes, then the other, underwear stripped down and off, brought to the tub, one foot in, water hot, hot, hot and foamy, other foot in, a hand in the small of your back, guiding you down into the welcoming water and you relax into the suds, hot on your buttocks, on your back, on your neck as the bubbles envelope you, lying back as the heat soaks into your bones and the cares of the day dissolve. Spray on, nice and warm, soaking your hair, shampoo rubbed in, scrubbed in, scalp tingling.

Arms lifted, scrubbed down with something rough and clean smelling soap, eyes closed, face scrubbed, then more rinsing, and you leave your eyes closed - it's easier that way. Leaned forward, then soap on your back and scrubbing in circles, top to bottom, left to right, rhythmically lower and lower, lean back, soap on your front, each breast lathered in turn, rough scuffs over tingling nipples, collarbone done, then ribcage and belly, one thigh up, scrub inside and out, top and bottom, do the calf, do the shin, do the ankle and foot, every toe, in between them, then back to the top and down the other side, turned over - it's awkward, suds on your chin while your backside is done, in between, rosy anus and vulva and clit. Back over again, and we start with the razor, from the ankle to vulva on left leg and right. Arms up, do the armpits, with attention to detail. From the start to the finish it must be done right.

Plug out, water spirals – stood up and you're dizzy. It's the heat, so you're held. Now sprayed down, pink and clean. Needles of water, just the right temperature, a thousand little pinpricks, reviving your skin, cascading down to the drain - hair soaked down, water streaming over your face, down your back, arms up and rinsed top and bottom, breasts and back and belly rinsed, nipples

The Bath

tingle under the jets, bent over, buttocks rinsed, anus and vulva, clitoral hood lifted and sprayed, and you feel the pleasure but not long enough, not nearly close to long enough. Stood up again, legs rinsed, back and front, each foot, each toe, behind the ears, under the armpits, everywhere with no spot missed. One step, two step, out of the tub and onto the thick bath mat, the room still steamy and hot, tropical and lush. Towels fluffy and warm from the dryer, and you're scrubbed down as you were washed, as you were rinsed, hair and face, neck and back, breasts and belly, backside and in between, slippery there, and sticky, and wet again as soon as it's dried. The warm towel down your thighs, down your calves to your feet, lift one, lift the other, ticklish as they're dried between each toe.

You're aroused now, but languid - will it happen, won't it? It isn't up to you, and it doesn't matter. Wrapped in another towel and lifted, carried out of the bathroom into the cool of the hall and the warmth of the bedroom, lying down on black sheets, crisp from the laundry, tucked in covered, face down.

Hands on your shoulders, slick with cream, rubbing steadily, deeply into the muscles, neck and temples, scalp and cheeks, then down your arm to your hands, rubbing the palm, coating each finger, then back and across your shoulders to do the other side just as steadily, just as completely, then up and down your back, slowly, slowly, and up over your ass, nothing missed, spreading your cheeks, into your anus and vagina too, very thorough, very businesslike, no moaning is permitted, no squirming accepted.

Strong hands kneading, moving down one thigh, steadily, slowly, strong hands kneading soft skin and firm muscle, down your calf to each foot, just a little ticklish but still no room for squirming from a good girl. Back up, over your ass again and this time your vagina is positively soaked. Spreading it, rubbing it, inside and out, little clit standing hard and your hips can't help moving though that isn't allowed either, and the hands move down your other thigh to do your other foot.

Then we turn you over and back up, around the front of your hips and over your belly, up your ribcage to your breasts, first one, then the other but not the nipples, no not the nipples, though they're standing rigid now, begging for attention. Only after both breast are smooth and creamy and well rubbed do they get their turn, rubbed and tweaked but still not enough, not nearly enough, and they are aching, bursting for attention as the hands slide up to do your collarbone, your neck, your throat, your chin, your cheeks.

And now we're done, languid, squirmy, time for sleep, no more touching for tonight, but naughty girls will sometimes touch although they're not allowed and so the collar is buckled on, the cuffs locked to it to keep you good, ankles together, chain run down to the ring at the foot of the bed, covers pulled up and tucked in to keep you safe, kissed on the cheek and a parting smile and whispered words, and then lights out sleep tight, tomorrow is another day. Rinse and repeat and repeat and repeat.

Part Two

Yeah I know you. I know everything about you. I'm not talking about the details, the trivia doesn't concern me, but I know everything that matters. I don't know what you do but I know you're good at it. I don't know your name, but I know it's a name that counts. I don't know where you are but I know where you're going, and that's up. Fast. You're top of your class, top of your program, top of everything you turn your hand to, and nobody ever sees your secret doubts. You've got style and taste and everybody wants to be seen with you, though really they have no idea who you really are. And right now you're wondering how I know all this and it's very simple. You're reading this and this is part two.

So there are a million copies of this book out there, and a million women have picked it up. And most of those who've read part one just don't get it and they've already put it down, and of those who get it most can't take it, can't deal, find it too strange, too scary, too intense and they have put it down too. And the largest group of all just hasn't bought this book, because good girls don't read books like this, do they?

But you're here, you get it, and though it's very much new and even slightly scary it isn't too intense, no not at all. You want more, you're eager for more, you can feel the need for more in every nerve in your body. And we already know you're not a good girl. No, you're a woman and the feelings in your body right now are anything but girlish, though this part so far is pristine clean, nothing here to shock your mom or break your so-styled image.

But what matters here isn't what's said but what's about to be said, and you know about that, just like I know about you, and that's why you feel that tension in your belly now, that anticipation. You understand what's happening here, and you want it. You want it intense, you need it that way and it arouses you so much to think that you just might get it that you can't think about anything else but what we're going to do in part two. We've begun now, and though you don't know how far I'm going to take you, you know you need to find out. Look at the door, wherever you are, look away from this page, look at the door. Do it before you turn the page. *Now.*

Part Two

Done it, and realize that you have, quite deliberately, come through that door, picked up this book, turned the page. You have chosen this road, started the journey, our journey, and you can't pretend to be innocent this time. It takes a certain kind of woman to take this little challenge you didn't know you were taking when you picked up my words. It takes a rare kind of woman.

And that's how I know you, because I understand the kind of woman you are. You're smart enough that you've yet to meet a situation you couldn't handle, you're driven enough that you're used to coming out on top. You're accustomed to being in control, and your problem isn't finding a man, it's finding a man to meet your standards. And that's exactly why you're reading this right now - alone with me in your bed, on your couch, where-ever your are right now with time to spare, time to share what we're going to share. It's just you and me and our little exploration, our secret journey into the untrespassed sanctity of your secret inner world. And secret is the word, honey. This isn't the kind of book you read in the park, on the train, or in the lounge by the airport gate. This is the kind of book you read in private with one hand, and it's the kind that's going to stay in your mind long, long after you're finished, after we're finished. I can make you only one promise honey, at the distance in time and space that separates you and me right now, and that is that you're never, ever going to forget what you're experiencing here, and you're going to spend your nights dreaming about it, dreaming about me, dreaming about us. So make sure you've closed that door behind you, honey, make sure we won't be disturbed, because I have plans for you. The journey has begun.

Yeah, you already know what's happening here, or at least you think you do, and the difference between you and all the others is, you're still reading. They can't handle what this interaction is going to be and you can. Or at least you think you can. Or at least you can't say no to the challenge, and that takes a woman with all the qualities I just listed. So yeah, I know you. You can't say 'No', to challenges, can you? It isn't in your nature. Your instincts just react like that, make you try to get the upper hand in any situation, in school, in work, in life and oh yes with men, especially with men

Yeah, I haven't seen your face, haven't seen your body but I know the way men look at you, turn to watch you walk by, every one of them so eager to get close to you, do you favours, give you presents, touch you briefly on the hand. They want to do it just in case that makes you like them more, refusing to believe they haven't got a chance. You know what they want, and that makes it so easy to get what you want from them. You don't even have to manipulate them, though I know you're good at that too. Yes, you're good at games like tease-and-leave, good at maybe-later, good at look-but-never-touch.

Men are toys for you, so much fun to play with Christmas morning, but by New Year's Day you're bored and they're broken, tossed aside, forgotten for the next one. And maybe you should feel guilty about all the hearts you've

The Secret Journey

shattered but the hard part is getting them to give it up so you can just move on. And like I said, you're not a girl, not anymore, you're a woman, and it should come as no surprise you're getting bored with toys, correct me if I'm wrong. Yeah, you get what you want from them but you don't get what you *need*, that's something else entirely. You need to be challenged and that's exactly why I made this challenge. I know you can't say 'No' to it, and so the only word I'll take from you is *"Yes"*, and *"Yes"*, and *"YES!"*

And yes, your breath is starting to come faster, because you know I have what you need. What you need is where I'm taking you, on this secret journey to the dark side of your mind. Think about that for a moment, and think about your body. Think about why your lips are dry, why your heart is beating faster, why your crotch is getting damp. We still haven't shocked your mom here, honey. But you know what's going to happen, just like I know you. You know I'm going to take you just the way I want to and you know you can't say 'No'. Not to me you can't, you couldn't if you tried, though because you are who you are you'll try anyway, just to see if I let you get away with it.

So I'm not going to let you get away with it, honey. We already established that back in part one. "Yes" is your word, your only word, between these sheets, between you and I. "Yes" is your word, and you're going to say it now, say "Yes" for me. And you can't help but say it.

"Yes", silently, subvocally, barely parting your luscious lips but still moving them. Moving them because you have to, to make this as real as it can be. Moving them because I want you to, and because you want so much to be mine.

"Yes."

And yes, I know you. I know exactly where you are right now, in your mind, in your body. I might as well be watching you, watching you read this, watching this start to turn you on. That excites you, doesn't it? Excites you and scares you too, and you can feel me right there, can't you? You can feel me in the room, feel my eyes on you, focused on you, reading your thoughts before you think them. You can't help but wonder where I'm watching from, and though you know it's impossible you still feel it, still feel me there. And you can't help but look around the room to see where I am.

Go ahead, look around, check the door you closed behind us. You can't see me, but guess what? I *am* watching you, right here, right now, as I write this, as you read it. I can see you, oh so clearly, see your breasts, soft and firm and tempting, see your legs, your thighs, your round, inviting ass. I can see your lips, already parted, watch you lick them. You're proud of your body, but it makes you shy to know I'm watching. You want me to like it. I can see your eyes, see them flutter, see the shyness that you haven't felt in years. You're a woman but being watched like this makes you feel like a girl again, brings that rush to your stomach.

Part Two

Remember your first crush? Remember the long nights, wondering, dreaming, wishing? *Does he like me? Does he want me?* I can see the little tremors in your throat, in your hands, I can hear the catch in your breathing. It turns you on to know I see you and you want me to be turned on by the thought of seeing you naked. And yes, honey, I'm going to see you naked because you're going to strip for me, you're going to show me everything, one piece at a time. And you're going to make it good, make it slow, make it sexy for me, yes you are.

So say it for me "Yes, yes, *YES*!" You know what I like to hear.

"Yes," and we'll release your body, free your flesh from its confinement.

"Please," and we'll release your soul, turn you into purified sex.

Say it. "Yes please, let me strip for you." Nobody's watching but me honey, that's why I had you close the door.

"Yes please, let me show you everything."

Nobody's going to know what you're doing here, honey, nobody but you and I. So take your top off, slowly, slowly. Do it, really do it, before you read another word. Do it now. Right now.

Part Two

Good girl, so sexy. Now get your tits out, firm and full Are your nipples hard yet? Not as hard as they're going to be. Do you wear a bra? Let's get that off too, reach up, snap the clasp, shrug it off. That's what I like to see. You have such lovely tits, honey. Show them off for me, hold them up, offer them, rub them, rub them hard, squeeze them. Remember last time? Remember how they felt, remember how you felt, squeezing them for me, pinching your taut, tight nipples, holding them up for me?

Let me tell you about your breasts, honey. They're beautiful, womanly, and they're so much you. I don't care if they're big or small, what matters is they're warm and soft and curved and ripe. So stick them out, show them off, prove you're a woman, show them to me, shake them, wiggle them, make me want them. Oh yes oh yes, feel them move when you breathe, deeper now, and faster. Feel them ache for my hands. Your breasts are meant for my hands. Imagine for me now, imagine sitting on a pillow on the floor, leaning back against the luscious couch, leaning back between my legs, snuggled back with my hands on your breasts from behind, rigid nipples sticking out between my fingers. That feels good, feels intimate, feels warm and safe and close and right. It feels right because it *is* right, because that's the way it's meant to be.

You're the woman, I'm the man, and my hands belong on your body. That's the connection, our connection, our little private secret. You offer it and I accept it, simply, naturally, as easy and refreshing as cool water on a hot summer day.

And there's still nothing here that would shock your closest friends, though now you might not choose to share with Mom. But your friends aren't here and Mom is a long way away and right now it's just you and me, and what I want and what you need. And I don't want your tits anymore, honey, I want your ass. I want to feel it, firm and round and swelling. I want your belly, so smooth and rounded. I want your long, firm thighs, honey, so get your clothes off, get the rest of them gone, pants off, skirt hits the floor.

What kind of panties do you wear? No, don't answer that because I don't care. Underwear is a highway sign, interesting only because it tells you how close you are to where you want to be. So get rid of them too, honey, if you had any on to start with. Panties off, and are you wet beneath them?

Slide your hand down to find out, and of course you are, you've been wet since we started part two. You've been wet since you picked up this book. You've been thinking about it constantly, if you've even managed to put it down, it's been in your brain, in your mind. Every time you go through a door you go through our door, every time you see something written you're reminded of these words. It makes it hard to concentrate, doesn't it, honey? It makes it hard to get your work done when all you can think about is what I'm going to do with you next. Go on, ask for what's next. Say "Please," you naughty little girl, all wet and naked and so turned on.

The Secret Journey

"Please."

"Please," comes automatically now doesn't it? "Please" slips so easily from your lips. "Please, take me, please fuck me, please use me." Say it honey, say it right now.

"Please, take me, please fuck me, please use me." And now you're going to show me just how much you need it. "Please, take me, please fuck me, please use me."

Now stand up, legs apart, stick your ass out, stick your tits forward, lips parted, make it good. Do it, really do it, honey, because it's what I want you to do. Stand up, legs apart, present yourself while you read. And you know what you're asking for here, don't you honey? You're asking for my arousal. You're on display now, showing it off for me, showing me that *yes*, you are a woman, *yes* you are *my* woman and yes, yes, *yes* you are going to give it all to me.

You're saying, "See what you do to me, see what I'll do for you."

You're saying, "See what's yours, take what's yours."

Yeah, you want me to want you, you need me to want you, and honey you're getting your wish because right now there's nothing in the world I want more than you, and the only reason I'm not fucking you already, not slamming it into you so hard you think the world will end, is because I want to string it out, make it last. I want to see, want to know, want to *feel* just how much you're mine. Legs wider now honey, do it for me, feel the moisture on your cunt. Legs wider, ass out further, tits out further, and it's getting difficult to read, isn't it? Just a little awkward here, and you can't believe you're doing this, but you're doing it, spreading yourself, posing for me, this man you've never met. Not met yet, anyway. *Yet.* There's promise in that word. Does that excite you honey, the thought that maybe one day our journey will bring us together?

That's up to you and it may be true, but it's also a question for tomorrow because what matters right now is legs *wider*, bent right over, ass right up. Bend way, way over, feel the stretch, feel yourself open up. Can you still feel my eyes on you, honey? Legs wider still, do it, do it now, and you'd better find something to brace against or you're going to fall right over. And we can't have that, can we honey, because then you couldn't read, could you? And we very much want you to savour every word, every moment, every breath, every heartbeat of your time with me. So get yourself in position on your bed, over your desk, against a table, anywhere, I don't care. What I care about is legs straight, legs spread, ass up, bent right over with your eyes locked on this book and your cunt throbbing and juicy and now it's opening for me, all by itself. Arch your back, you know the way, make it good, make it hot, make me want it. Do it, fucking *do it*.

Fuck that's hot, honey. And now just think about how you look. Think about my eyes on you, drinking it in, narrow waist and flaring hips, breasts

Part Two

pointed at the floor by your tight and rigid nipples, your graceful slender neck, your soft hair and your ass, oh yes, oh yes, it's all about your ass, upturned and inviting, spread and vulnerable and offered up like ripe fruit. Feel my eyes on it, on your swollen cunt, on your stiff little clit, rigid now, peeking out from its cover, eager, oh so eager to be touched, rubbed, pulled, pinched. Imagine the effect on me, how that talks straight to the back of my brain, straight to my cock. You need my words, but what I need from you is pure body language, pure female sexual invitation, pure ass wiggling, cunt spreading, wet, musky, eager desire. You need my words, but what I need is your sounds, your moans, your groans, your desperate, pleading screams of sexual need.

You know what I need so talk body language to me, honey, ask for it with your ass. Make it say "I need you to fuck me."

Make it say "I'll be anything for you, your woman, your slut, your dirty little flirty virgin, or your easy, eager whore."

Make it say "I'm yours, all yours. I'll do everything you want just so long as you do it to me, and do it hard, and do it fast and make me feel it, make me take it, force me, fuck me, use me, abuse me, do anything, do everything just at the end just please, please fill me up to overflowing. *Please* spray me, *fill me,* drench me, drown me in your white hot juice."

Yeah honey, work it. Work it hard while you devour my words, let me see it, hear it, feel it. Work it so I have to watch, so you own my whole attention.

Yeah that's the way. And I'll bet you didn't know your ass was quite that eloquent but it is. It sends that message to a thousand men a day, and nine hundred look and look away before you catch them and ninety try to date you up, and maybe nine have ever really touched you, but there's only one whose ever made you feel quite like *this* and that's me and you haven't even met me. Yet.

Yet. There's that word again. It implies a future, but this journey we're on is a long one and right now is right now, and what I want *right now* is your pretty little cunt, petals spread wide, glistening, open, eager, inviting. Just slide a hand down there and do it honey, feel it open up for me, feel how swollen it is. You can't help but slide a finger over, slide it up, slide it in. You can't help but fuck yourself as you present yourself for me, bent over, open, willing, wanton. You know I'll like what I see, and you do like to put on a show, don't you honey?

Yeah, show me; hump it, do it, in and out and in and out, faster, faster, harder, and deep. Oh my God that's good, honey, that looks so hot. You didn't even know you had this in you, but I did. I do know you, and you understand that now, you get the picture - well part of it at least. Think about how you look there, one hand on this book, this thin thread of connection from my mind to yours, and the other on your pussy, finger fucking yourself to turn me on.

You didn't forget that part, did you - that you're doing this to turn me on. You didn't lose that point in your eager, slutty self-love, in the one woman orgy you're putting on right now. You didn't forget the point here is for you to please the audience, like any performer, and yeah, you're putting on quite the performance right now. The only difference is, this isn't play acting, this is as real as it gets. Go ahead, fuck it harder, you know you need it. Are you moaning yet? Are you tearing the breath from your throat in gasps as your clit swells and longs to burst? Think about that word – 'yet', think about how much more real this is, how much more intense, more passionate this is than simple boy-meets-girl. Think about how you're giving yourself now like you've never given yourself before and think about how you want to make it even more real, think about how much more you need.

And you need a lot now don't you honey? Hard and fast and deep, so do it, fucking do it, take it, grind it, get into it, show me just how slutty you can be. Get it off for me, harder, faster. Scream for me, beg for me, arch for me. "Please," remember that word?

"Please fuck me, please please *please*." Say it honey. Say it again. Loud.

"Please fuck me." Louder.

"Please fuck me." Louder still.

"Please fuck me, please fuck me, please make me take it, hard, hard, hard."

So yeah, I'm fucking you, I'm fucking you deep in your dirty little mind, deep in all those dark fantasies that have never seen the light of day. That's the most erogenous zone of all, and I'm fucking you hard where it counts.

It's getting closer now, your screaming release, your offering, your gift to me. It's coming up fast, so legs wider, ass higher, cunt up. Spread for me, open it up and make it happen, rub it, fuck it hard and harder and you know how hard it makes me to watch you, know that this very second you have me absolutely rigid, cock stiff-solid, straining, bursting and it's all because of you. Yes you, right there, right now are doing it for me, right here, right now. You're doing it for me with your hot little pleasure dance. So think about me right there behind you, watching this, and show it off for me. Show it good honey, make it good, make it dirty and beg for it, show me your orgasm is going to be all for me.

"Please, can I come for you?" Say it. Say it loud, no holding back.

Say it again. "Please, can I come for you?"

Say it louder, and make your ass say it too "Please, please can I come for you?"

Plead for it. "Please I'll be so good for you."

"Please, I'm giving you everything."

"Please, I'm your good girl."

Convince me that you need it, and maybe I'll let you.

"Please, let me come, let me come, let me come."

Part Two

Or maybe I won't let you. I bet you never thought of that, honey. I bet you never imagined I might stop and leave you hanging, leave you right there on the edge, just to prove I can. So think about it, while you rub your clit, while you ride the edge, think about it and wonder what's going to happen next. You'd stop if I told you to, yes you would, because that's the nature of the game we're playing here. You'd be swollen and pouty, and oh, so frustrated, but you would stop, you'd do what I told you because you don't want to break the spell. You need this and yes, you want to be a good girl for me. Good girls do what they're told, don't they? Don't they? Say "Yes," for me, honey.

"Yes, I'm a good girl." Out loud.

"Yes, I do what I'm told."

Good girl. So now that we've got the rules established, now that we understand each other, you're going to get a little treat for being so obedient. Remember that good girls do what they're told. Remember that, know it, feel it in your soul, and say it again.

"Yes, I'm a good girl."

"Yes, I do what I'm told."

And now I'm going to tell you what to do and that is come. Come now. Right now! Now! Come hard, give it up for me, pound your cunt, pound your clit and come until you scream, long and loud enough to scare the neighbours, pump your hips and you can't stop, do it, do it, do it fucking doit *doitdoit*.

Do it until you can't any more, until you're a limp, sweaty, trembling mess, lying there exhausted, slumped in disarray, nothing left of the poised, in control woman who turns a thousand heads a day. Nothing left of the organized, in charge, self-possessed woman everyone knows. Nothing left but sex, dripping from your well used cunt, throbbing through your swollen tits. Nothing left but full, flushed flesh, mind too far away to even read this clearly. Breathe deep honey, breathe deep and feel me there with you, smiling, touching, caressing. Breathe deep and let the walls fall down, feel so safe here alone with me. Feel your pounding heart slow down, feel yourself relax, just slide down where you are and smile. That's the smile I want, satisfied, womanly, taking pleasure in knowing how much you've pleased me.

That door we've come through is closed behind us now, closed so far behind us and we're moving forward, moving forward, into the place you need to be. You're moving on the journey, down the road, just floating down it with no effort at all, watching your old life slip away, becoming who you really are. Just feel me there, feel languid, lazy and you're going for a quick nap, nothing wrong with that now. You'll sleep the sleep of the well serviced woman, the good girl whose given it all and taken it all.

So feel my arms around you, feel me close, see my eyes on yours gazing deep, two inches away. Feel my lips on yours, so close and comforting and gentle. Feel me there, and know I'll still be here when you wake up, still watching you, watching over you. Have your little sleep, warm and safe and sated, smiling gently in your fulfillment. Ready? Feel your breathing slow, feel the relaxation. Feel me there and close your eyes at the end of this sentence, close them right now.

The Trainer

I look for posture first. Some look for size, some look for form, but I want winners, and thoroughbreds will lie to you with either. Look at how a colt carries itself, that's where the truth is. Watch for the skittish, indifferent or hostile - that's not a horse to work with. Watch for the colt that meets your gaze, that stands its ground, assesses you, comes to see what you are. Size and form don't make winners, spirit and courage do. You have to know how to judge winners. I'm a trainer, that's what I do.

Women are no different. This one wore clothes of casual style on a firm, athletic body, but it was her posture that drew my eye - upright and confident, shoulders square, back straight, neither flaunting her breasts nor hiding them. Her walk was an easy stride with a natural roll to her hips, and she navigated the crowd by the betting windows as though entitled to the space they gave her. She was a thoroughbred. More than that, she was a winner. Her spirit showed. She met my gaze in passing, gave me the same dismissive look she gave a thousand men a day. A woman like that draws notice, and she hasn't got time to invite attention from every idle gawker. Cut them down fast, get on with business is her automatic reaction. I held her gaze, watched her eyes widen at my impertinence, then narrow in warning. I cocked an eyebrow, watched her response, watched her blink and look away, and then she walked past as though she'd never seen me. I smiled to myself. I'd be seeing her again.

I turned back to watch the start, the business at hand. Aurora Australis was running this one, with Lacey Dubois in saddle. Aurora was a winner, an eighteen hand stallion who lived for the race. Lacey was not, despite her casual style and firm, athletic body, her posture gave her away. She was the owner's daughter, spoiled and haughty, and far too concerned with wresting daddy's attention from her over-competitive mom. Lacey was the wrong rider for a horse like Aurora, but that was a decision beyond my control. The bell went and they started well, running hard in front of Red Rocket. It was the race Aurora was born to run, with a hard charging rival and victory in his teeth. By the first turn he had a head. By the back straight he would have had half a length on his own, but Lacey went wild with the crop, broke his rhythm and it was neck and neck. Rocket crowded her and she lost her nerve. Aurora sensed her uncertainty and he slowed in response. In the last turn Rocket slid in front, then Miracle Worker hemmed them in from the side. Still Lacey drove him, though the race was now over, there was nowhere for them to go. At the finish they showed, behind Miracle Worker by a head. I nodded, made notes. It was what I had expected, in outline if not in detail. Aurora ran best when given his lead, and Lacey was not one to do that.

"Did your horse win?" It was the woman, it hadn't taken her long. Dark eyes and dark hair, pretty features, no hint of uncertainty shows in her voice as she approaches the stranger I am to her. She's used to being in control, this one.

"I don't have one running."

"But surely you bet." Her look is arch. She's deciding if she'll bet on me.

I shake my head. "I never gamble."

"So what are you doing here? I've seen you before." Her curiosity is genuine.

"I'm a trainer."

She hesitates, eyes widening just a touch. She hadn't expected that.

I smile. "Wait there, please." I point to one of the stadium seats in the aisle behind me. Her face shows confusion, then challenge, then acceptance. She drops her eyes and turns to sit down. I return my attention to the track, as the next set of horses parades past to the gate. I watch their postures, watch their gaits. These are my rivals, my competition, and it is important to know where they stand. I can see her reflection in the glass barrier in front of me, sitting awkwardly, uncomfortable. She's unused to this sort of situation, unused to being in less than total control. She doesn't like waiting there, but she knows what she needs. And so do I.

The bell rings, the horses run. There is another winner, and more losers. I study form, make notes, mark two late runners who show hidden potential. It is the last race, and the crowd rises at the end, the lucky heading for the payoff windows, the rest filtering back to the stairs, to the parking lot, to the lives they'd come here to forget for awhile. A couple of desperate losers pick their way through the discarded tickets that litter the floor in the faint hope of finding an overlooked winner. The woman is still waiting, my eyes meet hers, and she gets up to follow me. I head for the door that reads No Entry. Down the stairs are the stables, smelling of hay and horse sweat. Jack Dubois was waiting there, his face tight and strained. Behind him Lacey was leading Aurora into his trailer. I couldn't see her face but I could tell from the stiffness in her back that there had been a fight. He ignored the girl behind me, launched straight into his speech.

"I expected a win."

I met his gaze. "I only train the horse, Jack."

His jaw tightens, then relaxes, and he turns to look at his daughter. "I know..." there was resignation in his voice. He seemed about to continue, then became aware of the girl. "We'll get Aurora put away, you go on ahead."

The Secret Journey

I nod. "Good luck, Jack." I train for Jack Dubois by choice. I could make other choices, and he and I both know it. He has no choice but to deal with his selfish daughter and ill tempered wife. If he had been a different man he might not have had a problem. He's wealthy, old money in shipping, a force to be reckoned with in the circles where power counts for everything, and he knows better than most what a fortune won't buy. He's asked me to teach Lacey to ride, but what she needs to learn can't be taught in the saddle. She's just not a winner, and I don't have the time to waste trying to make her one. I didn't envy Jack.

I turn to go, the girl follows, out to the parking lot into the cool night air. I open the door of my crewcab for her, enjoy the brief touch as she brushes past. Her jeans tighten over her trim backside as she climbs up and I smile. Nothing wrong with her figure - for the rest, we would see. I close the door, go around and get in. She gives me a smile as I buckle in, nervous and suddenly shy. It takes courage to do what she's doing, courage and faith in her own sense of judgment, to get in a truck with a stranger like this. I start the engine and pull out, heading away from the crowds, away from the racetrack's blue-white floodlights, into the moonlit darkness, its secrets and its promises. I switch on the radio to spare us the small talk - find music, dark, rhythmic, compelling. Is she thinking about friends she ditched at the track, her boyfriend waiting at home? Is she thinking of me and what she is doing? Her eyes are on mine when I look in the side view mirror. In the cab's close confines I catch her scent, the warm, rich tones of female arousal. She wants me, wants what's about to happen, and it shows. We travel down the gravel concession road, pass farms set well back, most dark at this hour, a few showing lights. I turn into my own lane.

I think of my living room, hard wood floors, fine wine, good music, the rug and the fireplace. I think of seduction, of caress, exploration, excitement, new intimacy. That's not what she's here for and tonight is not that easy for either of us. I open the door for her, see her nipples tight against her shirt as she climbs into the cool night air. Crickets sing spring-mating love songs in the long grass, and amorous frogs answer from the pond. It's warmer in the barn, from the body heat of a dozen horses and the insulating hay piled high upstairs. The smell is earthy, familiar. The hands have been and gone, the stable cleaned, the horses fed and watered. Alec the barn cat yawns from his throne on the shelf beneath the heat lamp, granting me passage into his domain with a flick of his ears. I take her into my office, close the door.

"Here." I take her hands and see the reaction in her face. It's the first time we've touched and she's wanted that awhile, wants more now that she has it. Her fingers are small and delicate, and I pull them across my desk to grasp the other side. "Keep your hands here." She doesn't question, doesn't struggle, just does it. She's bent at the hips in this position, her perfect backside perfectly presented for anything, everything I want, and yes, I want it, want it all. I nudge her ankles, move them shoulder width apart. I could take her now, and I very much want to. But it isn't time yet, my day's not over and she can use the wait. The key to training, horses and dogs, cats or women, is patience. She's taken a risk, now she needs to know she judged correctly, needs time to settle into this new role she's found herself in, that neither of us imagined when we set out for the evening races, a thousand years ago. I sit down and do my paperwork, log my race results, plan the training for the week. She watches me with interest, grows bored, looks around the room, bookshelf and books, framed pictures, riding tack on pegs. I concentrate, but I can't help but be aware of her firm, round breasts moving with her breath, her scent mingling with the smells of the barn. Soon. Very soon.

I finish, stand up, she looks up at me. "Did you forget about me?"

I meet her gaze. She doesn't want control back but she'll take it if she can. That's her instinct, she can't help it.

"No." I take a length of cord from the wall, coarse and functional, watch her eyes widen. "Put your hands behind your back."

She hesitates. She has to make the decision. If her courage fails it's over, right here, right now, to end in awkwardness and a long cab ride. Neither of us wants that, but is she brave enough?

She is. She holds my gaze, straightens up, slowly slides her hands behind her. Only then does she look down. I smile and move behind her, take her wrists and figure eight the rope around them, one, two, three, wrap the crossover, finish with a stop knot. She's breathing faster now as I undo her jeans, slipping them down to her ankles, dark thatch of pubic hair showing through sheer panties, wet in the middle. They're plain, solid coloured, comfortable, casual style. They suit her.

"What's your name?" I push her forward, guide her until she's bent full over, cheek against the cool oak desktop.

She tells me. There's a catch in her voice as she says it.

I smile as I pick up my leather work gloves. Like her underwear her name fits her well, both feminine and practical.

"Are you ready?"

"Yes." She can barely whisper it.

I nod, though she can't see that, pull on the gloves, rough leather, worn smooth in the centre. Her buttocks are smooth, invitingly curved. I pull her panties into the middle, pull them tight so the bunched fabric splits her cunt, the swollen, glistening lips swelling up around it on either side. She gasps at my touch. One hand in the small of her back, raise the other, pause a moment to see the anticipation in her face, bring it down hard, hear the smack, see her jerk and quiver, hold her still. Raise it again, bring it down, steady, rhythmic, over and over. An involuntary cry escapes her lips as her ass blushes red for me. I watch her face, set now with determination to not give in to tears, to not give in to me. She's fighting it and it's hard for her. It would be easier for her to just surrender, but she can't, she has to be brought there and there's only one way to do that.

I keep up the rhythm, feeling the exertion in my arm now, feel her buttocks growing warm even through the glove. She bites her lower lip, her eyes misting. It hurts, and it's humiliating and that arouses her which is more humiliating still. I watch her fight it, watch the struggle, feel the impact of her flesh beneath my hand. Every smack brings a wince now and she shakes her head unconsciously, trying to ward off the surrender we both know is coming fast.

It would be wrong to say she liked this, though there's no question it arouses her. No more than I like putting her through it, though the strain of my cock against the denim of my jeans proves the deeply sexual nature of the act. It's necessary though, and bonding - the foundation for the structure we're going to build. What shape that will take is an open question right now, but our future stretches beyond this moment, this night, and because of that we must play out this duet to its finale. And there is a moment when she hangs there, the silence punctuated only by the steady slap of leather on flesh, and then it comes, her face relaxes from resistance to acceptance, her lips parting, her eyes growing heavy lidded. Ever so slightly she arches her back, presenting herself now, opening herself.

She wants to be fucked, she's so ready, slick hot, reduced to her cunt and its need to be filled. I continue the rhythm, continue the tempo - she'd take it right now anywhere she could get it, in her mouth, in her ass, if that's what I wanted. She's achingly empty and yearns to be filled, overflowed with my lust. She's rocking her hips, gasping for air. She needs it and so do I, my cock filled to bursting, rigid now, and heavy, as eager to fuck her, to take her, to make her, as she is to have it happen.

Without even trying I'm spanking her harder, the slaps sound like gunshots in the confined space. There's nothing I want more than to impale her, hear her scream as I drive deep inside, to conquer her, over and over again, make her beg for it until she can't even speak. There's nothing I want more than to empty myself into her, flood her cervix and womb and body and soul with everything I have, everything I am.

But I can't, and I stop, take a long moment to steady myself, lost as I am in the drug that she is. She's different, this one. I want more from her than I can say, more than I have from all others who've crossed my life before her. Is it only because she has so much more to give? And if I'm to have her, have her completely as she completes me, she must learn who I am, who she is, how we fit each other as no others do. Ride a horse too soon and you'll spoil it. I knew her potential the moment I saw her. She doesn't know - not all of it, not yet, but she will very soon, because I'm going to show her.

So I take off my gloves, and slide down her panties to join her jeans around her ankles, and revel a moment in the heat of her ass. Her cunt glistens, swollen and sticky, and I slide a finger into her, feel her arch back and moan. She's ready, so ready, and I slide the finger out and up again to her anus, slide it in, hear her gasp, it's so degrading for her to be used like this, probed and inspected like this, but she needs it and so I'm giving it to her. I hold it in her and she humps back, humiliating herself further in her heat. She wishes it was my cock violating her like that, and one night it will be, but not tonight. No, not tonight, and I slide my finger out of her again and she moans in frustration.

On the wall is a harness made not for a horse but for a woman, bit and bridle of leather and rubber coated steel. I take it down while her eyes follow me, bring it to her. Her lips part automatically and I slide the bit between her teeth, pull her hair through the leather straps, cinch it tight. It's uncomfortable and she instinctively tries to expel it, but of course it doesn't move. The collar is next, thick leather with a steel ring in the front to take a leash. She doesn't struggle, doesn't protest, just accepts it as I lock it around her neck. She'll take a leash tonight. She'll take much more. Her lesson is about to begin.

I stand her up and look at her. Her shirt is pretty, a white cotton blouse and I tear it open, buttons popping to fly around the room. Her nipples are just that hard, popping little buttons, painfully stiff and I indulge myself with her teats, pert and firm, upstanding little mounds, weighing them, squeezing them. I twist her nipples hard, watch her eyes as it gets painful. She pleads with them, pleads for it to stop, pleads for it to be harder. I give it to her harder, hard enough that my fingers hurt and she moans, but she takes it. Of course she takes it. She needs it and she knows it. She has no idea yet just how much she needs, but she'll learn.

I'm going to teach her. I'm a trainer. It's what I do.

Part Three

So that's my little tale of the racetrack, honey. Did you like it, did it arouse you, turn you on? Did you wish you were that girl, wish you could be taken like I took her, just abandon yourself, feel that vulnerable, take the risk but know that it's safe? Did it make you breathe hard, make you squirm, make you wet? Did you play with yourself while you read it, rub your hot little clit just because it felt so good? Did it wrench an orgasm from your womb, or did it get two? Or more? It made you keep reading, I know that much.

So here's the catch, it's a true story - or at least it's truly a story and I'll let you decide what's truly the truth. She's just like you, her name is yours, and you're both caught in this hazy world of words, caught between reality and imagination. She was my muse, and I touched her just as I am touching you, but the difference is she broke my heart. And you might find it amazing that a woman half imaginary could do that, but she did, just as you might yet. She was so beautiful it hurt, and so she wounded herself in the mirror. She was stormy as a lover and yes I loved her stormily though I never heard her voice except inside my mind. All writers need a muse and she was mine, perfect in her imperfection and no less real for being ethereal.

But she's the past and you're the future. You're real, I know you are, because you're right there reading this. You picked me up in the bookstore and you bought me coffee when you bought this book. That was date number one, honey. Ten short minutes of talk-and-tease, the kind of interaction whose only real purpose is the only purpose you won't admit to, which is to determine if you want to fuck this stranger you've only just met, and to induce me to want to fuck you too. And when that worked you took me home, coffee forgotten, focus on the real purpose, which is the kind of sex that comes from instant chemistry, ab initio sex, wet and wild with the thrill of discovery.

I showed you the door then, you know the one. Look at it now, right now, look up at it and then look back to this page. That's the door I showed you, the door you came through, the door that started you down the road. You stripped for me, showed me the dirty flirty girl behind that in-control image, showed me the inner slut, the depraved and desperate need that lurks just below the surface. You put it on the line for me, gave it all up and that takes a certain amount of courage, honey. That's where you found out that yes, I really do know you.

Part Three

And now you're back again, the door closed behind you, and our journey before us. Soon we'll be in that place where self revelation happens, in that languid time after the violent need of fresh new sex, lying, sweaty and sated, tracing a finger idly over heated skin, asking those casual questions whose answers mean so much. "So what are you thinking?"

But we're not there yet, not yet, and right now all you're thinking is, "What is he going to do with me this time?" The answer, honey, is anything and everything. Yes, you're ready for it, ready for more and we're going to pick up right where we left off.

So let's go back to last time first. Part two, remember that? Remember the scent of your cunt and the smell of your sweat, remember how it felt to offer yourself, open yourself, reveal yourself. Remember immersing yourself in your own sexuality just because it turned me on to see you do it. Remember being on display, bent over, ass up and cunt open. Remember your arousal, your heat, your raw and burning need. Remember your orgasm, wracking your body, tearing out the centre of your soul. Remember being that exposed, that raw, stripped more naked than naked. Remember your own sounds in your ears, moaning, groaning, screaming. Remember your voice begging for it, pleading for it, "Yes," and "Please," and "More." Remember how much you gave me, how much you gave yourself in giving me, and remember the way you felt at the end, languid, relaxed, post orgasmic, warm and safe and drifting off to sleep.

Remember that, because I remember it. That's burned into my mind now as strongly as it's burned into yours, and I'm never going to forget it, and neither are you. Remember that and then we'll start, and this is a new game, the game called part three. Another little twist and we'll learn another word. And first I want you naked. Yes, I want you always naked, naked is your place when you're with me, so get your clothes off. Off! Do it fast, do it like they're on fire, rip them off, tear them off, pop the buttons, burst the seams. Get naked, get raw, don't ask questions just do it. Do it. Do it. Book down, just drop it. Do it, do it now.

Part Three

Done it. Good girl. So now I want you kneeling down, back straight, head level, lips parted, and you already know what this is going to be about, don't you? Really do it, don't just imagine it, get on the floor, on your knees, ready to please. Do it, honey, because you have to do it for this to work. Nobody's watching, it's just me and you so do it, fucking do it. On your knees for me, because that's where I want you, and right now that's where you belong. Don't turn the page till you're there.

Part Three

And now you've done it and you do know what's coming next, making your mouth water and your lips part and your tongue slide nervously over your teeth and yeah it's making you wet. It's making you wet because I'm making you do it. You know what's going to happen, honey, but not yet, not yet. I have something to teach you first. So last time I wanted everything from you but right now all I want is your focus, your attention and nothing else. So focus close, let the world fade away. I'm right there with you once again, but even more real this time, and you're going to have to work for that. So close your eyes and feel me there for five long, slow breaths, call up the image in your mind, me standing right here in front of you. Close them now and count.

Part Three

Open again, and here I am. Look up, hold my gaze now, look into my eyes, feel them open you up. Hold it longer, feel me take you, feel me possess you, kneeling there, looking up as I'm looking down, drinking in each other. Feel the connection, feel the power, feel the surge and the swelling emotion. You're mine and you know it and I know it and that's the way it's meant to be. And now that we've established that, we can begin. You're going to learn about me.

So look down, start at my boots, look them over, check them out. Women always look at shoes, so see what you can learn from mine. They're basic black, solid and practical, boots built to get the job done, but burnished bright enough to see your image there in the high-gloss polish. Absorb that lesson, think about what it tells you about me, then let your eyes slide up to my five-oh-ones, clean jeans, well fitted. Keep them in mind while you keep moving up, over my calves, over my thighs, feel the desire to touch, to explore, but no, honey, right now it's look-but-don't-touch. You know that game, don't you honey? How many men have you played that one with, and now you're on the other side. Not getting what you want feels better than you might have imagined, doesn't it? It's nice, so nice to not have to make decisions for a while.

Slide your eyes up higher, up to my hips, to my belt and, oh yes, to that oh-so prominent bulge behind the Levi's patented button fly. Feel your mouth water, feel your eyes get big as you take it in. If we were in public you'd just steal a glance, and you know you're good enough to not get caught. So we aren't in public honey, and this is about learning so take it in, every swelling curve of it.

Oh yeah, you long to touch now, you can feel it in your fingers, that twitchy desire, to touch, to feel, to explore right there. I have your focus now, honey. You want to feel it stiffen and swell beneath your fingers, to know that it's you I'm responding to, to know what you're arousing, what you're unleashing when you indulge yourself in my cock like that. Feel your desire in the way your body leans forward all by itself. You have to tell yourself to keep straight, to hold back, because you want to show me you can do that, that you can play this game, do what's expected, do what you're told, be a good girl. It's easy to do what you're told when it's what you want to do, that's all you had to do in part two, but it's a little harder when what you're told and what you want are different things. Oh yeah, you want so bad, so very much, to just reach out and touch.

But honey, I have faith in you. I know you'll do it, be so good for me. So just look, and if your nostrils flare as you try to catch the scent of masculine musk, well, you can get away with that, I didn't tell you not to, did I? Smile the secret smile you smile when you get what you want by the back door. Smile that smile and inhale that scent that makes you so giddy, and so thoroughly wet.

Imagine nuzzling it, imagine the feel of rough/smooth denim against your cheek and the taste of the cloth, and the slightest hint of what lies beneath.

Feel your mouth water with desire, and swallow hard to keep control, and move your eyes up because you're still learning. Check the belt honey, basic buckle and hefty leather, basic black like the boots, wide enough to fill the loops. Are you getting the picture here? The theme is basic. I'm a very basic person. I'm not into flash, not into show. I'm into substance, I'm into real, which is why I'm in to you. Basic instinct, yours and mine, male and female, that's the way it's meant to be.

I know you, remember that? That was the lesson of part two. I know who you are, what you need, and this is it, exactly. Keep focused on the belt, honey, and think about why I choose to wear it. Imagine what it might be for. Imagine how it's going to feel against your cheek, and against your cheeks. See the shirt tucked in around it, heavy, pressed cotton, collared, buttoned, loose but fitted, as basic as everything else. Follow the buttons up over the belt, lean waist to wide shoulders to find my eyes again, still locked on yours, they haven't left since you looked down. Short dark hair and dark, dark eyes, back where you started, burning into yours, steady, hypnotic. Hold my gaze till you look down, slide your gaze back down to my belt, to my swelling crotch, that's where you should be looking, that's where your eyes belong.

Do you feel powerful here? Do you feel powerful naked while I'm clothed, kneeling while I stand, eye to eye with my thickening cock, wanting it and denied it. Do you feel powerful waiting to be told what to do, waiting for me to say yes or no? Or do you feel caught, helpless, heart beating wildly, desperate for release with nowhere to go, and nothing to do but wait.

Well, you should feel powerful honey, which doesn't mean your aren't helpless, captive and captivating at the very same time. Yes your heart is racing, and yes your knees are weak. Powerful doesn't mean you aren't frantic to get contact with my cock, doesn't mean you have anywhere else you can go and most certainly doesn't mean I'm not going to get exactly what I want from you, exactly the way I want it, how I want it, when I want it. But yes honey, you have power even though you're here to do only what I want. You have power, kneeling naked, because you are in this position more beautiful, more desirable, more fundamentally female than you have ever been before, freed of every last inhibition, the single, focused object of my unslaked desire.

Because while you wait for me to say yes or no, what do you think the chances are that I'll say anything but yes? What do you think the chances are that this little encounter is going to end any other way than exactly how you're imagining it right now, with your lips wrapped around the base of my rigid, thrusting cock, with my hands tangled in your hair, pulling you onto it, fucking your mouth like it was your cunt. What do you think the chances are that this will end any other way than with my sperm squirting over your face, your lips, your tongue and right down your eager, hungry throat?

And isn't that exactly what you want, what you crave, what you need? Do you imagine I have any choice but to take you? Any option but to make you mine in exactly the way you need to be mine? You have power here because of who you are and what you are, the quintessential woman. All that counts right now is your mouth and my cock, and you can felt the heat coming off it even through my jeans. Move your cheek closer, feel that warmth and look up, meet my eyes again, plead with them, beg with them, make me know there's nothing more you want in the world than to put your lips on my cock. See my hand reach out to your hair, feel it tangle tight, feel it pull you closer, firmly, slowly. Feel the touch of the denim, just the way you imagined it, rough and smooth, with that throbbing, solid presence swelling just beneath. Feel your heart beat faster now, feel your breathing quicken, your nipples stiffen, your clit get hard as your cunt gets wet.

Rub your cheek against it, feel that heat. Lick it honey, lick the cloth, suck against it like you could suck that throbbing shaft right through the fabric. Feel it stiffen more as I pull you tighter. Get your face in my crotch, inhale that scent. Make me promises with kisses, feel your power as you hear me growl.

That's the way bitch. *Bitch!* Do you like it when I call you that? Do you find that degrading? And if you do, does degradation juice your cunt? Ever see a bitch in heat, honey? Ever see a real bitch, down on all fours, ever see the way she gets her haunches up, flips her tail aside so the alpha wolf can fuck her till he's done? Bitches in heat have no shame, no inhibitions. Bitches in heat exist to get fucked. That's just like you right now honey, so maybe you like to be called bitch and maybe you don't but it's an accurate analogy so that's what you're going to be until we're done.

Suck it bitch. Suck it hard, and by now the wet spot on the front of my jeans is getting big, and it's time to get my cock out, get on with the job. Feel fingers tighten in your hair while the other hand undoes my belt buckle. Hear the jangle as it comes undone. Pop, pop, pop as the buttons come open, easy access, imagine that. Underwear out of the way and there it is, honey, there it is, bitch, right in your face.

Long and thick and hard, your holy grail, your heart's desire and you know better than to waste time getting it in your mouth. Hefty is the word, a cock big enough you know you're going to feel it take you, feel it deep, feel it hard. Rub your cheek against it, kiss it, get to know it, you're going to be getting very familiar with it. Feel the texture, silk-soft over solid steel, kiss it, lick it, taste it. Yeah taste it, there's that musk you scented before, so rich, so strong. Flick your tongue over the tip, over the slit, then slide your lips down, slowly, slowly, make it good.

The Secret Journey

You're wrapped around it now and your first inhale is so full of man-musk that it nearly makes you faint. Do you like it, bitch? You don't need to answer, not that you could if you wanted to now, with your mouth stuffed full of my cock. I can hear it in the way you moan when you get your lips around it. I can see what it does to you by the way you latch on, slip your tongue around the taut-swollen head, by the way you slide forward, take it in like you were starving for it. And you were starving for it, weren't you bitch? You *are* starving and now I'm feeding you, and you'd say, "Thank-you, sir," if you could but you can't say anything with my shaft in the back of your throat, so just show your appreciation with your tongue bitch. Make it feel good for me, because that's what you want. You want me to feel good, right, bitch? So good I shoot my load down your hot, eager throat. Feel it fill your mouth, pushing in, almost too big to take.

Both hands back in your hair now, pulling your head back and forth, bobbing you up and down on my cock like some kind of sucking machine. *Take it bitch.* Take it hard and take it deep. God that feels so good, and you have to understand how it makes me feel to have you kneeling for my cock like this. It's intense, it's powerful, as powerful as every thrust that forces your mouth open, hits the back of your throat.

Am I pulling too hard on your hair, bitch? Am I going too deep, too hard, too fast? It doesn't really matter, because all you're going to get is deeper and harder and faster from me, bitch. Let's make the term a little more accurate. *Cocksucking bitch.* How does that work for you? Just think about the way you look right now with your lips stretched tight and your cheeks working in and out as you bob your head on my cock like you needed it for basic survival.

Easy little bitch. That's accurate too. Yeah, you're so easy for me. You, get wet with a word, go down with a glance. *Hot little bitch.* And yeah, you're hot honey, there's nothing hotter in the world than you kneeling there sucking like your life depended on it. Watch me fuck you bitch, watch my muscles tense and clench, shoulders tight, pulling your mouth hard onto my cock. It hurts when I pull your hair but you don't care, you just need to get more cock fucked into you, forced into you, you're all about the big splash that's about to happen, the one gun royal salute fired straight into you. You swallow, don't you bitch? You do now, let's put it that way. You're going to swallow every drop, except what gets sprayed across your face.

Hear the slither as I pull my belt out through the loops, long and thick and shiny and black. Does that give you a rush, bitch? Does that make you suck a little harder, a little faster, just to show me how eager you are to please? Did you figure out why I wear it yet? You can see it now in the corner of your eye, doubled in one hand while the other stays in the back of your head, setting the pace, urging you on. Feel me stiffen, get harder, longer, thicker. Sense my balls tightening up. Come on get me off, bitch, cocksucking bitch. Come on do it,

Part Three

fucking do it. Taste the precum, bitch, leaking from the slit, flick your tongue over it and moan in desire. *How about it bitch?* You ready for it, ready for the spurt? Put your hands on my ass bitch, feel it flexing, thrusting, riding your face. Feel the muscles clench rigid, feel my cock swell to bursting, it was big enough before, fucking huge now, swollen and slick with your saliva. Take it bitch, fucking take it. You can feeling the steady throb, taste the stream of precum, a steady flow now, rising to the final flood.

Look up into my eyes, bitch, beg me with them, beg me for the finish. Hear me grunt, an inarticulate animal sound as I fuck you faster. You've done this to me, reduced me from words to noise, made me want you, need you, more, more, *more*.

Yeah I can feel it now, building up inside, getting ready to burst. You're going to get your wish, bitch, going to get it good and hard. You make me so fucking hot, and with one hand I'm ripping my shirt open, sweat gleaming on my chest, then both hands back in your hair to keep you right where I need you, force you on and off my cock like the dirty cocksucking bitch you are.

Your jaw is aching now, you've held it wide so long, and your scalp is sore where your hair has been pulled, and maybe you even want it to stop. Too bad bitch, ride it out, take it like a good girl because that's your role here, that's your only purpose, this moment, this instant there's nothing in your world but my cock. It doesn't matter that your jaw hurts and your lips are bruised. This one isn't about you, it's all about me and the only thing I'm going to do is fuck your face till I unload.

Oh my fucking god, you look so good with those big, big eyes pleading oh-so sweet, and the sweat is beading on my skin with the effort, salty, musky, and male, all male. See my face contorted, hear me grunt, see my shiny, sweaty body tense hard-hard-hard and then I roar and that's all it takes, spurting, spraying, jetting sperm, down your throat, in your mouth and overflowing, and I'm still thrusting in, in, in, *in*! Feel it drip over your chin, over your tits, feel my cock come free and spray your nose, your cheeks, your lips, and in again to finish. Feel it pulsing, throbbing, fuck that's hot. Feel me stagger, feel me put my weight on you.

And feel the throb in your cunt now bitch, *well used bitch,* feel your clit rigid and wanting it, feel your pussy clench just like it was what just got fucked, got filled, got flooded. Feel your orgasm right there, so easy, one touch and you'd fucking lose it, scream and writhe.

But guess what bitch, you don't get that this time. This time is about me, remember that? This time is about my cock. Your time was last time honey-bitch, and this is this time and this time you don't get to get off, soaked and eager as you are. This time it's my orgasm and not yours and all I'm going to do is fall to the bed because my knees are now too weak to hold me up. I'm going to flop down and pull you down with me, under the covers so you can curl up in the crook of my arm. And I am going to put my arms around you, twine your legs in mine, so that I know exactly where you are. Yeah, I can feel your sperm-wet face against my chest, I can see your big, big eyes looking up into mine. And I'm going to pull you tight, close-tight with too much strength because my co-ordination is gone. And you are going to squeak and purr and cuddle tight and it feels so right that you're still drenched in my cooling, drying, sticky juice. And I am going to smile and lean down and kiss you gently, taste the last trace of myself on your lips. And then I am going to do the man thing, which is close my eyes and go to sleep, because you've done this to me, taken everything I can give, drained me dry. And now it's your turn to watch me, hear my breathing slow down, feel the steady thud of my heart against your cheek. Yeah, you can watch me, and you can know you've drained me, emptied me, gutted me, know that I have given you absolutely everything, my body, my spirit, my soul.

Yes honey, I have spent myself on you and in you in the most absolute sense. And you are going to know that I am now yours as much as you are mine. And your arousal is going to fade to something warm and close and caring, something more tender than you dare to say. So feel me there, so close and warm, male to your female, yang to your yin. Feel that all is right with the world, as we take another step down our road. And you are going to watch me for a little while, and then you'll be asleep yourself.

The Traveller

Tokyo to Moscow, Moscow to London, London to Toronto. Sometimes I feel like I live in airports, my world reduced to an ever-changing, never-changing vista of departure lounges and baggage claims. My services are specialized, and when they're needed, they're needed immediately. When I'm lucky that means corporate air, more often it means I'm on the next commercial flight. For this flight there was nothing left in the forward cabin, so I'm in the back with the tourists.

It really doesn't matter. The trivial comforts of first class can't offset the fundamental realities of air travel, the unending line at customs, the inevitable delays, the hour or five or twelve spent sitting there at thirty thousand feet, while the plane flies and the passengers while the time away with a book or the inflight movie. I bring my laptop when I fly, and try to get done the work that must be done before I land. It's just part of the job for me, but still I love airports, I love the potential they represent, all those distant destinations, a million people mixing and moving. Anything could happen, and life still holds surprises.

I know the drill at security, carry-on baggage on the X-ray belt, laptop out of its case, phone and pager and keys in the plastic bin, take off my belt and put it in there too, so the buckle won't set off the alarms. I stand in line, go through the metal detector, get waved on and collect my belongings as they come through the X-ray. My belt is what matters this time, solid leather, thick and black, not really dressy enough to go with my tailored suit but I don't wear it for show. This time they don't make me take off my boots, gloss polished, another minor departure from corporate image that has nothing to do with image. I go to the gate, board the flight and then we're flying, four hundred tons of jet and five hundred souls, hurtling through the sky at six hundred miles an hour. It's basic physics, the transformation of potential energy into kinetic, a modern day miracle, made mundane through sheer familiarity.

Just imagine what DaVinci would have given for the chance to see clouds from above. I ignore the view from my window seat, and concentrate on my laptop. I'm to be met at the airport, to finalize over dinner a transaction worth more money than the average man earns in a lifetime. It's imperative that I get it right; my only stock in trade is my reputation.

The Traveller

And as we climb away from the airport I find I can't focus. Corporate deals are something else grown mundane through sheer familiarity. I look at my archive of electronic mail, bring up one in particular. All it says is - *I'll be waiting.* I hold up my glass for the stewardess, a pretty blonde with a flirtatious smile. She fills it with red wine, and I admire her ass as she goes back up to the galley. She wouldn't mind if I asked her what she was doing after the plane lands but I'm not going to do that, I already have another plan. *I'll be waiting.* Such a simple phrase, but it sends a thrill through my body. *I'll be waiting.* It's basic chemistry, the transformation of potential energy into kinetic, an ancient miracle, but this time it's neither familiar nor mundane. I wonder what she'll look like, this woman I've never seen. I wonder what she'll *be* like. Unconsciously my hand moves to my belt. She'll be feeling it, in something under six hours, she'll be learning what I'm like, and she'll be learning what she is. I close the laptop and turn my eyes to the clouds, shaping them into whatever I want them to be. *I'll be waiting.* I don't even know her name.

Not soon enough the plane starts down, the wheels come down and we're on the ground, at the terminal and I'm walking into arrivals, about to present my best guess rather than my best work, an unforgivable sin brought on by my sexual distraction. Dinner drags as we discuss the frantic details of a deal gone sour. My clients smell of desperation as I lay out their options. It's an unfounded fear, they have nothing to lose here, but they're terrified of what they might not gain, the petty insecurities of small men with large wealth.

A rational analysis of their situation would put them beyond such concerns, but they are paying me for corporate guidance, not personal enlightenment, and so I keep my opinions to myself. I want the meeting to end at eight and it drags to nine, to ten, to eleven as I patiently unravel layer after layer of hidden agenda. *Will she be waiting still?* I think she will, but I won't know for sure until I get there. At last we reach the end, my best guess having proven correct, my best work proving unnecessary. Their driver takes me to my hotel, I check in, and check to see if the extra keycard has been taken. It has. I take the elevator up, go to the room, and take a moment to steady myself. *Deep breath in, deep breath out.* My erection strains against my zipper, in anticipation of what I might find. I slide the card into the lock, and open the door.

She's there, and I smile with satisfaction, and with desire. I don't know what she's told her friends and family, to explain her absence this night, but that doesn't matter. What matters is, she's there, waiting, just as she's supposed to be, black top, short black skirt, black stockings with the seams running straight up to her garters. She's waiting just as I told her to wait, kneeling on the floor, lips parted, blindfolded, hair in a ponytail, head down, hands held in the small of her back. Her nipples are rigid against the thin fabric of her conservative white blouse, and she's trembling in her excitement, barely able to breathe. Her knees are apart, exactly as expected, and as I come closer I can tell that she's been kneeling like this, and aroused like this, for the entire duration of my over-extended business dinner. I can tell because there's a thin, glistening strand dripping down from beneath her skirt, dripping down to join a slick puddle on the floor between her knees. The scent of female desire fills the room. She's such a slut, kneeling three hours to present her body to a stranger, with her anticipation, her excitement growing with every beat of her heart.

I stand in front of her, take her by the ponytail, move her head up, move it down, move it back and forth. She doesn't resist, in her current state of arousal I doubt she could even articulate the concept of resistance. She's here to do whatever I want her to do. She's here so I can shape her, into whatever I want her to be.

The first shaping is to establish the proper form of her relationship with my cock. I pull her head forward, turn it to rub her cheek against the hard bulge behind my fly. She moans in response. I let her feel it there for a moment, and then turn her back so she's facing it, her nose just half an inch away. She can't avoid its scent this close and her response is automatic, unconscious. Her already parted lips widen into a lush, receptive 'O', her dainty red tongue comes to moisten them in anticipation of what's about to come. I feel her pull forward, ever so slightly. She's eager to touch it, experience it, explore it, and explore herself at the same time, so the first lesson is in control. I relax my grip slightly and allow her to come forward until her lips just graze the fabric. She shudders when they do. Could it be that she came, right there? It doesn't matter. I pull her back, just a fraction of an inch and she makes a small, inarticulate noise of frustration, tugging forward against my restraint. She's waited so long, she doesn't want to wait any longer.

But she's going to have to. "Do you want it, cunt?" I ask her. She tries to speak and finds she can't, and I get a barely perceptible nod. *Cunt*. She understands the importance of the word. *Cunt*. That's the only name I know her by. She has another name of course, the one used by her husband, her friends and family, for the entire rest of her life. I have no desire to intrude there in the slightest bit. To know her name would be to elevate her from the status of *cunt*, and neither of us wants that.

I hold her head where I want it to be long enough for her to relax, to stop pulling against me, to accept that she's going to get it when I'm ready to give it to her. She's learning that what she wants, or doesn't want, has nothing to do with it, and that's an important lesson. I wait that long, and then a little longer, watch as she licks her lips again, her breathing quick, and as I watch she swallows nervously. I smile. She's going to learn to swallow too.

My cock is bursting, and what I need more than anything is to see the swollen head sliding past those red lips, see it glisten with her saliva, see her taking it, deeper and deeper. I reach around with my other hand, unzip my fly.

The Traveller

She jumps at the sound, instinctively starting forward again, but I pull her back, hold her in place with the swollen head of my cock half an inch from her lips. Her nostrils dilate as its musk fills her world.

"Tongue out, cunt," I tell her. She obeys, shuddering as it touches my waiting cockhead. Her tongue feels so good, so very good that it's all I can do to not shove the whole hard shaft down her waiting throat. With an effort I hold back, and slowly bring her mouth forward. She explores the head with her tongue, and finds the silver drop of precum at the tip. She licks it, savours it, swallows it, and I groan involuntarily. Yeah, she's getting to me, and she's going to get it in return.

"Go on, ask for it."

"Please…" Her voice is a trembling whisper, her lips grazing my cock as she speaks, every touch swelling it stiffer.

"Please what?"

"Please… please I want it… please…"

"What do you want?"

"Your cock… Please, fuck me with it, fuck my mouth with it, anything, only please…"

I thrust forward, forcing her mouth wider to accept the head, cutting off her words in favour of a more direct demonstration of her desire. Her lips close around the shaft and then she's sucking it, my hands gripped tight on her ponytail to pump her head up and down, enforcing her cock-submission, probing for the back of her throat.

She knows just what to do, my eager little cocksucker, using her tongue, using her lips, doing everything she can to get me off. She can't beg with her voice now, but she's begging me every other way, showing me just how much she needs this, needs to be on her knees like this, blindfolded, controlled, forced to accept my cock wherever I want to put it. She needs to be put in her place, in a way that absolutely no-one in her life has ever done. She needs it, and I need her to need it.

I pull her off, pull out, once more letting just the head graze her lips, and she begins begging again, immediately, instinctively.

"Please sir, come in my mouth." She licks the head, teasingly, almost playfully. "Please sir, come on my face." Her voice is insinuating, pleading.

I put my free hand on my cock, still holding her head right where I want it to be. Her words are quieter now, as if she's praying directly to the cock that's dominating her.

"Use me, please use me, humiliate me, anything you want, just please, please come on me, I need it so bad."

I pump my rigid shaft, feeling the tightness build up in my balls as she begs for it, as her lips and her words coax me to her own degradation, as my muscles stiffen and my cock swells harder, harder, harder still until finally I can't help it and I give her exactly what she wants. I grunt, forcing my cock forward, and torrent sticky strands of sperm to coat her cheeks, her chin, her lips, her tongue. The world goes dark and my knees buckle with the force of my orgasm, it's all I can do to stay standing as my hips pump my cock back into her mouth, finishing the last spurts there.

She swallows, of course she does, and then I'm standing there, breathing hard, looking down at her still parted lips, sperm dripping down her face to fall and mingle with her own juices on the carpet. I breath deep to recover, and then, still holding her ponytail, I guide her down, down, down, until her nose is right in the puddle. She gasps, her face flushed, more humiliated than ever, forced to confront the evidence of her own arousal like this.

"Lick it," I tell her, and she does, tentatively at first, her delicate tongue darting out to the scented juices soaked into the carpet. "Go on, show me what a cunt you really are."

She gets more enthusiastic, lapping eagerly at the fabric, sucking at it, smearing her face on it. My cock instantly hardens again, just watching her. She's going to be taking it again, and soon, but there's a second shaping to be done right now, now that she understands her role with respect to my cock. There's a chair behind me, and I let go of her ponytail and sit in it, watching her dirty herself. I put my boot down in the puddle, smear the toe into the stickiness and wait for her to find it with her cheek. She hesitates.

"Go on," I tell her. "Don't stop." A quick motion unbuckles my belt, and I slide it out through the loops, an unmistakable sound. She knows what will happen if she stops, but she doesn't want to stop, she just needs to know that she has to keep going. She hesitates another moment, and then groans, in arousal, in humiliation, and she continues licking, up and over the juice coated toe, her tongue working the polished leather. She's learning her place now, learning where she belongs, abased at the feet of a man strong enough to put her there. I still don't know her name, but I don't need her name. She's been reduced to *cunt*.

"Faster, cunt." She shudders at the word and responds to the command automatically, her tongue moving quickly, leaving the leather glistening in its wake. The shaft of my cock is rigid again, thrusting up through the custom-cut fly of my custom tailored suit. It turns me on to degrade her, and maybe there's something wrong with me but at this point I'm far beyond caring. It's time to fuck her now, and I grab her ponytail, pull her up, turn her around, bend her over the arm of the chair.

"Spread it, cunt." She does it, reaching her hands back, fingers finding her swollen flesh, parting it to show me the hot pink tunnel, wet and waiting. I nudge my cock against her slick-slippery slit, then thrust it in with one solid shove. It's tight, painfully tight, and she screams in pain and pleasure and climaxes right there as I pump her deep. "Take it, cunt." I spit the words through clenched teeth. "Fucking take it." And she does take it, she has no choice, it's what she is, and all she is. She takes it as my hands dig into her hips, as I force her legs wider, as I pound against her cervix. She takes it as I fuck her, make her beg for more even as I give her everything, over and over and over again. Her ass is so gorgeous, curved, female, presented, and the sight of her pussy stretched obscenely around my cock is sex itself, purified, concentrated, served raw and hot. My shaft glistens with her juices as she grunts and groans and begs for it harder. I tear a climax out of her, once, twice, three times, and watch her tight anus contracting hard each time. It makes me even harder to know that I'll be fucking her there too. She keeps on coming, keepings on taking it for what seems like forever, until her groans are as much from pain as pleasure, until she's sore, until I'm sore, until I'm done and my own orgasm hits and my balls contract and I empty them deep, deep inside her. She comes again when I do, the hardest one yet, her cunt spasming hard, her body shaking, screaming and arching, pushing herself back against me to get it all, get everything I can give her. She takes it too, and in that moment she becomes her cunt, becomes herself, becomes mine.

A long, long time later, we're lying together, her back against my chest, my arms around her, my hand cupping her breast, my cock still inside her. "I'm flying to Berlin tomorrow," I say. "I'll be back in a week."

"Mmmmm." She sighs and snuggles her backside back into me. "I'll be waiting."

Part Four

And will you be waiting, when I want you, honey? Are you waiting now? Let me set the scene for you, honey. Where I am right now it's summer, high summer. Where I am right now it's night, late night. Right now the stars are out and the air is warm and humid and ripe with expectation. I'm in the countryside and there's nobody here but you, you on the other side of this page, looking in as I look out. Right now the waves are lapping not far away, and right now you're on the other side of my door.

And I know you think I'm speaking in metaphors, but you're wrong, honey, I mean it very literally. There's your door and my door and we are exactly that close together. Outside my door is the road, and it's a completely ordinary road except for one magical property, and that is that it is a real and physical link between you and me. It doesn't matter where you read this, when you read this, when you go through your door, when you stand on the road, you're standing on a continuous ribbon of concrete that goes directly from me to you. Right now on my road there's a lone car coming, and maybe you're in it. Maybe you're going to go right past me in the next thirty seconds and neither of us will know. Maybe I'll be driving the next car you. The world is like that, full of small coincidences that you don't even know about until much later.

Right here on my desk is my phone, and if only I knew the digits I'd be dialing you right now. *Right now*. Think about that and listen for the ring. Listen for the ring and feel your heartbeat jump up a few notches as you do. Punch a few numbers and you'll be talking to me in seconds. We could be touching in under twenty-four hours, that's the magic of the modern world. We are that close honey, so very, very close.

Is it real for you yet? Is it real enough? Do you understand what's happening here? You and I exploring each other, and if I already know you because of what you are, who you are, who you must be to be still turning these pages, you're starting to learn something about me. You've got an image in your mind now, a very clear one. You're reading and I'm writing and in that process I am constructing thoughts in your mind. I'm building this world that you and I are sharing right now, and I can build it any way I want to. So what you have to ask yourself is - what kind of man builds his world this way? And to ask that question is to answer it.

Part Four

Yes, you're learning a lot about me here, more than my friends know, more than my family knows. Every word you read gives you another key to the darker side of my soul. That's something special, honey, that's something I don't give to many people. Women have come into my life, come into my bed, gotten close enough to know me very well indeed and yet they've never known this part. This part is something for me and for you and for nobody else.

And this part takes focus. Every breath I'm taking right now is going into my keyboard, into these words, into these pages you're holding right now. We're touching honey, we're holding hands. We're that close and we're at one of those delicate moments where words don't quite do the job.

Run your fingers over these words, honey. Feel their texture, feel the connection coming through, feel it soaking into to your pores. Hear the lapping waves, feel the steamy summer heat right here, right now. It's the same for me, because I know you're out there, I know you're reading this and I can see you right now with your eyes locked on this page and your heart beating faster and your lips parted. Feel your own breathing quicken to match mine. I can't predict the future honey, but I can promise you one thing, and that is that my words, will change you, have changed you, permanently. Whatever else happens, you are never going to forget what we're sharing here. And neither am I.

So I want to know you, honey. I want to touch you, physically, intimately. And the way that's going to happen is you're going to touch yourself. You're going to run a hand up over your breast and touch it the way I would touch it. Do it for me, honey. Do it right now, gently, firmly, amazed all over again at the warm softness of a woman. Does it surprise you that I can be gentle, honey? Does it surprise you that I would touch you with tenderness? Let me run my finger over your nipple, just enough to tease it to attention, let me marvel at your response, at your gasp, at the way your body moves involuntarily.

Lick your fingers and tease it with your slick finger tips, feel me kiss it when you do, feel the warmth spread through your body, feel my breath on your skin. There's something so special, so close about kissing your nipple. Offering a breast is such a maternal thing to do, it's *the* maternal thing to do, so warm and generous and right. Slide your hand to your other breast, tease that one too. Let me cup your treasures, let me appreciate the feminine wealth of you.

Lick your lips, touch them, run your fingers over them, feel me kiss you there, gently, gently, barely there. Let me make you want it, let me make you lean forward to be kissed, firmly, sensually. Feel me explore your lips. Yearn for it, feel your pulse pound in your throat. Trace your hand down, over your delicate chin, over your neck, back down to your breasts where your nipples are stiff and pointing, needing the attention back from your lips, slide your hand down further, ribs and belly, so soft and female, and let your nipples ache again with their need. Feel the swell and curve of your waist and hips, feel the round fullness of your delightful ass.

A woman is a beautiful thing, *the* beautiful thing, and you are a woman of infinite beauty right now. Run your hand down to your smooth, curvaceous thighs, feel the heat and humidity at your crotch as you go past it, feel your cunt swelling in response to your touch, to my touch.

Yeah, honey, this is what I want. I want my hands on your responsive body. I want to be looking in your eyes while my fingertips explore you. I want to drink every gasp, every motion. I want the sensation of your skin against my lips, firm and yielding. I want to scent the arousal wafting up from your moistening cunt, and I want the knowledge that your clit is stiff and getting stiffer, swelling in anticipation of the moment that I'm going to slide my hands right up between your thighs and revel in your wetness. That moment is coming, honey, coming soon, but not just yet.

First I want to kiss you, so turn your head to your shoulder and kiss it the way I would kiss it, gently, teasingly, inhaling your scent again. Feel it, feel my arousal at the wonder that is you. Kiss your arm, little butterfly kisses down to the crook of your elbow, give it little nibbles with your lips. Tongue the sensitive fold there, lick it, taste yourself, salty and fresh, and oh, so female. Do you know what it does to me to taste you like this? Imagine what it's like when you catch my scent, so fundamentally masculine, so powerfully directed at your most basic instincts, and you'll understand what your scent does to me.

And now, now is the time to slide your hand up to your hot, wet pussy, slide your fingers over your eager, pulsing clit and up in between your slippery folds. Feel the thrill, feel *my* thrill at your arousal. Close your eyes, picture your hands on my cock, feeling it swell, growing hefty under the weight of my desire. Feel the response in my groin as I realize that yes, I have you right here, right now, and yes, I want nothing more than to be inside you, deep, deep inside you, so deep it hurts, so tender it makes you cry.

So my instinct is to not waste time, to take you hard and fast, take you now, now, *now*, but I'm going to wait because this time isn't about fast and furious, this time I want to make you wait, make myself wait. This time I want to give you everything. So this time I'm going to rub my fingers, your fingers up and down your juicy, tight slit until you're going crazy for it, begging for it. Feel the pressure building up honey? Feel your hips starting to move all by themselves, pushing up, thrusting up to get more friction for your eager pussy. Slide those fingers past your clit and back again, and realize what a rush it is to have a woman like you, like this, getting hot and hotter for me.

Let me breathe you in honey, let me drink you, let me devour you. And bring your slick wet fingers up to your lips for me, honey, and taste yourself the way I want to taste you. You taste salty, slutty, sweet. You're sex distilled, bottled debauchery and I want every last drop of you. Do it again honey, scoop

Part Four

up your juices and suck your fingers, rub them on your lips. Do it again, and smear your face with your femaleness so when I kiss you all I can smell is your cunt. Do it again, baste yourself in your own juices, honey. Feel me kissing you, feel me needing you. Do it again, do it again, paint your tits with cunt cream, paint your nipples so when I suck them I can taste your sweet-sexy twat. Fingerpaint with fingerbanging, be my sex slut goddess, my sticky-girl muse.

Oh yes, honey, you are mine and I am yours, and I can't keep my hands off you. Give yourself up to it, feel my hands everywhere, feel the instinct that makes you spread your legs for me, spread them wide, you can't keep them closed. So spread them for me, spread them for you. Splay yourself, display yourself, reach down and separate your labia just because it feels so good to be open and feel me touch you there, so warm, so intimate. Feel me kiss your throat, watch me slide down to kiss your nipples again, tighter, harder than ever now, and sticky-slick too. Hear my breathing quicken as I lick them, as I revel in your feminine bounty.

Reach out and touch me, be bold, run your hands over my chest, over my abdomen, back down to touch my swelling cock again. Hold it, heft it, feel it and feel your response to it, so alive in your hands, getting bigger, heavier, harder just for you. Feel the need in your belly to have it in you. Hear me breath harder, hear me groan as you stroke it. Yeah I want you. You know I want you, and you want nothing more in this world than for me to want you more than anything. And yes, honey, yes I do want you. You can see it, sense it in the way I slide my hands under your ass and lift you, spread you like ripe fruit to be devoured. Feel the way your swollen vulva separates as your legs go up in the air, as I push them high and wide.

Reach down and spread yourself for me, pull your cunt open, stretch it wide, *wide*. Prove to me how open you are, and feel my hot breath on your clit in that endless, agonizing moment before my tongue makes contact. Feel the surge of pleasure as I lick you, stab my tongue at your eager clit. Do you want more of that, honey? Say yes for me, you know the way I like to hear it.

"Yes."

"Yes, please sir, please open me." Let me hear your desire.

"Yes, please sir, please make me come."

And you know I will because you know I love this, love giving you pleasure, as you give yourself to me. I love experiencing you at your most receptive, most feminine. You know I love to hear you moan, hear you sigh, so don't hold back honey, let me know I do it for you. Slide your fingers where I'm sliding my tongue and show me how much you like it. That's right, honey. Just lie back and let me make it feel so very good. Let me show you how much I want you, and that's very much indeed, that's more than anything. Let me taste you, let me see you let go.

You are right now the centre of my world, you are right now the most sexual thing alive, the most desirable, sensual woman that has ever lived and right now you are all mine. And what makes you that way is not just your hot body and not just the way you wiggle and gasp beneath my touch, it's more fundamental than that, it's you, it's the way you are, it's because you're the woman who has read this far, you're the woman who isn't afraid of my darker side, it's because you are the woman smart enough, creative enough, to turn these words into this complete experience. That's the rush for me, honey, that's what makes this work for me here in my sultry, steamy summer night. I know you're there, right there, on the other side of this page, the other end of this phone, the other end of this road, the other side of the door.

Yeah, you're real for me, honey, you're there and yes, you have gotten to the tender side of me, for just this instant you have tamed the beast. And yes, I'm here and my tongue is right on that magical spot, urgent, insistent. Yeah, I'm going to get what I want from you. And you are split, spread, swollen, slippery, so aroused you can't even think straight. So say it honey. Say "Yes," for me, say "Please," say those words, those magic words, over and over and over, say them loud, say them with every stroke.

"Yes."
"Please."
Rythmic.
"Yes."
"Please."
Steady.
"Yes."
"Please."
Harder.

Yeah, do it harder, honey, do it faster. Do it honey, and feel my tongue as you stroke your clit, ready now, feel the orgasm building up. Feel your womb get tight, feel your cunt throb, feel your clit swell to bursting. Just because it's tender doesn't mean it's not intense. Do it, honey, give it to me, legs spread wide and wider, get your cunt open, get your soul open, thrust your hips up, make yourself your own sacramental sex altar, let me worship at your temple, let me take you where you so much need to go.

"Yes."
"Please."
Say it.
"Yes."
"Please."
Stroke it.
"Yes."
"Please."

Part Four

Fuck it.

Oh yeah, honey. Harder now and faster. I want it for you so much, I'm going to make you come so hard, just let it all go because you can't hold on to it any longer, just let the pleasure sweep your body, let your cunt explode, just be it, feel it, do it, fuck it. Can you see yourself as I see you, like Eve, the original woman, the original beauty, passion made flesh and flesh made passion. Do you know how precious you are to me honey, do you know how much I need you right now? Come on honey, give it up for me, pump your hips, get your legs even wider and give it up. It's coming now, coming fast, your orgasm is there, right there honey, and it's going to happen right now.

Now! Now honey, release it, ride it, scream it out, let it consume you, consecrate you, purify you. And you are so beautiful like this, honey, you are my everything right now. Pump it hard, honey, feel the contractions, feel the rush, feel how right it is like this. You *are* your cunt now, honey. Feel the tingle in your nipples, feel the throb in your clit. Breathe for me, honey, in and out, deep and regular. God you are so beautiful. Breathe and feel it, shudder through it, buck and spasm. Be all woman for me, be all women. Show me how you are when you let go. Do it. *Now!*

Part Four

And when you're done, when you're finished, once every silver streak of pleasure has been milked from your contracting womb, once every last thrill and tingle has come through your body, then come down for me, honey. Let your body go limp, let your muscles relax and let me see you in that beautiful state of after-orgasm, your skin glowing, flushed, your eyes lidded heavy now in the aftermath, the smell of your sex filling the room. Breathe deep, honey. Let it wash you away, and you can lie there and feel me next to you.

Let me brush the hair from your eyes and hold you, honey. Let me lie with you a little while. Tell me how it was honey, and kiss me with affection. Let me talk about what I've learned from life, let me listen to your stories. Let me hear your heartbeat with my head against your breast.

Can I get you something, honey? Water, wine, milk or mangoes? Ice cream, whipped cream, or simply whipped until you cream? Pain or pleasure, lace or leather, tell me your favourite. Food, flesh or fantasy, there's nothing I won't bring for you. Are you still surprised, honey, that I can choose to be tender? I'm a real person honey, I'm more than just words on the page, more than just a cookie-cut character. I have depths you haven't dreamt of. Tell me your desire, let me make it real for you. Is it real enough yet? No, not yet, but getting realer all the time. You're still there and I'm still here, but we're getting closer. We're in no rush, honey, we have time, here in the private darkness of our steamy summer night. Here at the beginning of our road.

The Teacher

It's hard being a teacher, a high school teacher. What makes it hard is the girls, the women. When they start they're girls, gawky and shy, not quite co-ordinated, not yet comfortable with bodies which have transformed themselves in a few short years. They arrive as minor-niners with braces and bubblegum, playing dress-up with themselves the way they used to with Barbie. They giggle about boys, they flirt and fight and cry in response to floods of hormones they can't control, bringing on feelings they don't understand. They struggle through crushes and jealousies. They dream of their first dance, first kiss, first touch, first time. And then, a sudden four years later, they're women.

Young women to be sure, with their lives in front of them, but women, not girls. They know the power of their sexuality, and dress-up has been replaced with style. Their bodies are firm and lithe, fully formed and fertile. They know how to get what they want, most of them, and the ones who don't yet will learn soon enough. They are beautiful, in that first blush of womanhood. They are ripe, and they know it, and they advertise it to the world, knowing the wolves will fight it out to see who's going to win the prize.

Boys lag girls, it's just the way they're built. They come into school still children and when they leave they aren't yet men. Young women like older men for just that reason. They're attracted to maturity, experience, confidence, authority. Better to say they *respond* to such men. They can't help it, any more than men can help responding to women who are young and beautiful. It's not a choice, not an acquired taste, it's instinct. Basic instinct.

And if you're an older man but not yet too old, if you're fit and tall, if you're passionate about what you teach, if you connect with your students on their level, then it's inevitable that attraction will happen. I've had Valentine's cards appear in homework, answered the phone to silence and a giggle and the click-buzz of a hang-up, seen my name carved in a heart on the window ledge in the library. I've had secret notes mailed to my house and had other girls sidle up to tell me someone "likes me" in just that certain way.

It takes self discipline to resist when they sit in the front row, looking up at me with their eyes big, drinking you in as you stand there being mature, experienced, confident and authoritative. It takes more when they linger after class to ask a question, spark a discussion, share that precious three minutes before they have to run home to their private fantasy where the teacher/student veil is pierced.

It's just a crush people say, parents and relatives, friends and guidance counselors, as if that makes the emotions less important. That's wrong, so wrong. Emotions are emotions, and if crushes are fleeting, capricious, always ill thought out and often ill advised, they are nevertheless powerful. I used to say, "Just a crush," and sidestep the shy glances, the awkward advances. What else could I do? I dated women in my own age group, women whose sexualities are more advanced than kiss-and-fumble, women who appreciate the side of me that I keep strictly separate from PTA meetings and teacher's union working groups. And then Suzanne Smith killed herself on the last day of school, and her note told the world it was because she realized she could never have me.

A thing like that stays with you. Sue was quiet and studious and pretty, with a sly sense of humour that went beyond her years. It's the smarter ones who are most dangerous, the ones most likely to feel cerebral kinship across the generation gap. I teach creative writing, the last class of the day, and perhaps I should have recognized her attraction by the way she lingered afterwards to ask questions. Perhaps I should have seen it in what she wrote.

Her stories were longer than most, and far better written than even the average professional can produce. They tended to romantic themes. She left the last one she wrote in her locker when she went home that day of school, having cleaned everything else out. She titled it *The Millwheel*, a well crafted tale of a young woman and the miller's son, her secret lover. They meet in a secluded nook by the millpond, and though nothing more than a kiss occurs you can feel the passion lurking just beneath the words. Her parents find out and forbid her to see him because he is beneath her social station. She refuses to end it, and they arrange to have him drafted into the army. He goes to war and she waits, until news comes that he's been killed. In despair she dives into the millpond and swims until she's swept into the raceway, dragged down and under the churning wheel, killed in an instant. Her final thought is of her lover, her wish that his soul will return to his father's mill, so they can always be together.

I wept when I read her story, it was just that good. What I didn't know was that she'd written it for me, only for me. She had laid it all out for me, as plain as can be, and though I'm good at spotting student crushes I'd never even guessed at hers. She laid her heart before me, bared her soul, and what did I do? Graded it A+ in red pen and wrote 'Excellent work, Suzanne. The use of the millwheel both to symbolize life and to foreshadow of death is very powerful. Your characterization is beautiful. Best of luck in university next year.'

Suzanne never got less than an A. She had a dozen scholarships from a dozen top ranked schools to choose from. She could have had any career she chose, anywhere she chose, travelled, learned, loved, grown, raised children and grandchildren. She threw it all away because I didn't return an attraction I didn't even know existed, that I couldn't have returned if I had known. I remember the way she hugged me on that last day of senior year, the last day of her life. She held me tighter and longer than she should have, my first and last hint at what lay beneath her shy and quiet surface, and I kept my professional distance and congratulated her and shook her hand and wished her well.

Perhaps I gave her some paternal good advice, I can't remember. I do remember so clearly when her mother called. "This is Sue Smith's mom," she said, and then she burst into tears. Now I bring flowers to her grave every year. I kept teaching, what else could I do? I love my work, even when it hurts. I still get Valentines and carefully penned notes on purple stationary. I still sidestep them, but more carefully now, and with compassion. Never again have I said the words, "Just a crush."

Four Septembers after Suzanne, Julie arrived in that same class. She was tall and tight bodied, adolescent lean with high, firm breasts and long, long legs. She wore ripped jeans and torn t-shirts, and one or the other was always black, tight enough to show her figure, loose enough to show she didn't care. Her attitude towards school skirted the border between bored and amused. She tolerated the system because she had to, but she made it clear she didn't buy our line about how important the process was.

Julie was as smart as Suzanne or maybe smarter, but her work was habitually late and typically sloppy, though she'd throw in the occasional A+ effort just to prove she could do it, if she wanted to. Most of the time she read a book in class, making her own use of the time we made her spend at a schoolroom desk. She was a reader, gaining admittance through words to worlds she couldn't yet access any other way. She was doing what she wanted now, not waiting for some magical after-time, after graduation, after university, after landing the career, the promotion, the directorship. I had no idea what she did after school, no idea what her home life was like, but her writing spoke volumes, themed dangerous and dark. She sat in the back where Suzanne had sat in the front, and she never lingered to talk after class.

Until one day she did.

It was a Friday in early October, a cool and crisp day. The bell rang at four and the class evaporated in a babble of young voices. The usual handful stayed behind with questions or problems to address. I dealt with each one, made notes in my log where I had to follow something up. Julie was last in line.

"Julie." I looked up from my desk, gave her the standard quick smile of invitation to tell her it was her turn. She didn't say anything for a moment, just watched the previous student go out the door.

"Julie?" She was still watching the door as it swung shut again. The latch clacked closed, and then she knelt down beside my chair. "I want you to teach me, sir." Her voice was nervous, her face determined. She knew what she was doing, it scared her, she was doing it anyway.

The Teacher

My blood ran cold. On the surface it was an innocent enough thing to say. I am after all her teacher, and all my students call me "Sir", as they call all male teachers "Sir" and all female teachers "Ma'am". Completely innocent, except for the way she was kneeling, except for the tone of her voice when she said it, the way she emphasized "Sir", in just that way. She knew, somehow, and she was acting on what she knew to get what she wanted. I just stared at her, unable to speak until she said the words I dreaded, the words I somehow knew were coming.

"I was at the Club on Saturday night, sir. I saw you there." She put her hands behind her neck, fingers laced together, raising those high, firm breasts to me, offering them. I ever so carefully didn't look, but before I didn't look I saw her nipples, standing hard and proud, jutting evidence of her arousal. They weren't a good sign. She knew about the Club. *The Club* with the capital implicit. The Club was in the city, a good two hours from here. The Club was where my other life was lived out, in a world far darker than this quiet little community could ever imagine.

And here was Julie, little Julie. How did she... how *could* she know?

It didn't matter. "Julie, stand up." I said, in my best teacher voice. It brooked no misunderstanding or disobedience. I couldn't allow this to continue.

"Yes sir," she said, and stood, with her hands still clasped in the back of her neck.

"And put your hands down." I glanced out the windows, afraid someone might have already seen what she'd done. Innocence, in a case like this, is no defence at all.

"Yes sir." She put them down by her sides and stood there, obediently, quietly, waiting. She was doing exactly what she was told, which was exactly the wrong thing, under the circumstances.

"Julie," I said, my voice quieter. "This can't happen. You're too young..."

"I'm old enough, it's perfectly legal."

"I didn't say it wasn't legal I said you were too young."

"I'm not too young to be your student, sir."

"Not this way, Julie."

"In every way, sir."

"Julie..." I groped for words. "You don't know what you're talking about."

"Yes I do sir. I saw you at the Club..."

I held up my hand, my stomach tightening. "And how do you know about that?"

"I had a hunch. I went there. I saw you, sir."

"Enough! This isn't something we can do. We can't even talk about it. Ever." There was finality in my tone.

Julie looked at me, her eyes big and round, her cheeks flushed. There was a tremor in her voice. This had taken courage for her to do, I had to hand her that. She wasn't about to give up.

"My marks are bad sir," she said. "I want them to be better, I want to go to university. I need you to help me, to punish me when I'm bad, when I don't do my work."

"Julie…"

She didn't let me finish. "I'll be good for you sir, I'll make it worth your while. I promise. I'll do anything." Her voice was pleading, desperate for help, desperate for acceptance.

I looked away from her, looked out the window so I wouldn't see her tight young body or her big, begging eyes. I took a deep breath and swallowed. What she was proposing might be legal, but the school district has a single rule for a situation like this. *Hands off.* It was up to me to be the mature one, the responsible one, to turn away from what this beautiful, intelligent, eager young woman was offering, to refuse to give her what she clearly needed so much. Her parents, the principle, my colleagues, the world at large, they all expected me to make the right decision here, to live up to the expected code of ethical conduct, to not take advantage of the situation. Just as I had with Suzanne.

And would Suzanne be alive now if I'd kissed her, if I'd taken her, slept with her? Would she have enjoyed her teacher-fling and then gotten over it, gone on to her scholarships and her degree and her brilliant and successful future? Would she now be writing me a warm Christmas card, remembering what we had briefly shared, excitedly describing her new and expanding world? Or would it have ended in disaster, in heartbreak? It might have, but nothing could have been worse than what had really happened. The world at large didn't have to bring flowers to the grave of a smart young woman who'd died for unrequited love. I'd apologized to Suzanne's mother as though I'd done something wrong, and she'd looked at me and looked away and said "I wish…" She hadn't finished, but I knew what she was wishing. She was wishing I had loved her daughter, if only for a little while, and thereby saved her life.

I looked back to Julie, standing there, young and firm and waiting. Decision time and I really had no choice.

"Be at my place, ten o'clock tonight. Be on time or don't come. If you don't come, if you're not on time to the second, it's over." I looked her in the eyes. "Understand?"

She shuddered. Did she climax at that moment? "Yes sir."

I jerked my head at the door and she ran out, not looking back. As she grabbed up her books I caught a glimpse of what she'd been reading while she should have been paying attention in class. A plain black cover with a single red rose, I knew that book. How many young women had their first look into their own sexuality through the eyes of its thrice-tested heroines? I looked

The Teacher

down at my desk, put my head in my hands. *What have I gotten into?* It was wrong, and it would ruin me, but I couldn't deny my desire to bend that lithe body to my will, to discipline that brilliant, undisciplined mind. My cock strained upwards at the thought. I felt guilt and desire, fear and lust. *I can't do this.* The words ran through my mind in a permanent loop, but I was doing it.

Or was I? I hadn't expected Julie's approach, I had no plan to deal with it, but I'd made one on the spot. Ten o'clock was a deliberate choice, not so late that she could protest it was an unfair time to meet, but late enough that her parents might stop her from going out. My phone number is unlisted, my address along with it. Smart teachers do that, to cut down on the prank phone calls and the toilet paper strewn all over the lawn. Students have dug it out before and I'm sure they will again, but she'd have only a few hours. If she didn't figure it out in time I'd be able to end it cleanly before it began, save my career, save myself from the memory of Suzanne.

At home I made supper, tried to grade papers. Visions of her body kept intruding, visions of her in the same positions I'd had Lize in, had Jana in, had Colleen in at the Club. Beautiful women, intelligent women, women who came to purify themselves on the Club's altars of leather and steel, who came to consecrate themselves with me. The difference was, Julie was my student, forbidden fruit. That was exciting, in a way that none of the others could offer. That was exciting, as much as I wished it wasn't, and the danger involved was just the icing on the cake. Unable to focus, I tried to read and found no distraction, and found myself wishing I'd set the time for nine instead, to end the anticipation sooner. I didn't want her to come, and I wanted her to come more than anything. Finally I laid the riding crop on the desk, ready, and forced myself to do my own writing. Ultimately I managed to lose myself, to do it so thoroughly that when the door chimed I'd lost track of time. I glanced at the clock. 9:59 blinked to 10:00. Her timing was perfect. We'd play this game out to the end.

She was there at the door in a pleated skirt and neat white blouse, demure and conservative clothing, not at all like her usual style, and dangerously close to Suzanne's. I don't know what lies she told her parents to get herself out of the house. It didn't matter. I was in too deep to back out now. I didn't say anything, just turned and went back inside. I heard the door close behind me, the slight scuff of her shoes on the carpet. I led her into my study where I had been writing, where the riding crop waited. I pointed to the desk. "Grab the far edge," I said. "If you let go before I tell you, it's over."

"Yes sir." She bent over, stretched out, wrapped her fingers around the far lip of the desk. That position forced her onto her toes. Roughly I shoved her legs apart, so each foot was outside the edge of the desk, hooked around the legs. She inhaled sharply, her nose almost touching the riding crop. She had transformed in that moment, from girl to woman, her breasts pressed flat against the wood through her thin blouse, her legs long and feminine, her waist small and tight and her ass, her taut, rounded, upthrust and spread ass, so wonderfully presented beneath the skirt, ready for anything I might care to do to it.

I picked up the riding crop from its place between her outstretched arms and flexed it, watched her muscles tense in anticipation. I flipped up her skirt with the crop's tip. She had no underwear on, and her cunt was shiny wet, and swollen.

"You've been a bad girl Julie," I said. I raised the crop. "A very bad girl."

"Yes sir," she said, her breath catching in her throat. I brought the crop down, fast enough to whistle through the air, hard enough for the smack of impact to echo around the room. The stroke left a burning crimson streak across her smooth round buttocks and ripped a cry from her throat.

"You've put me in a very difficult position, Julie." I kept my voice level, in control, but I was angry at her. I was angry for the boldness of her action, for the inescapable logic of her proposal, for reminding me of Suzanne. I brought the crop down again, slashing it hard against the sensitive crease that divided her ass and her thighs. She moaned something inarticulate that might have been, "Yes, sir."

"Your homework is not up to standard Julie." Slash!

"Your attitude needs correction Julie." Slash!

"I'm not going to stand for this Julie." Slash!

At first she said "Yes Sir," after each statement, each stroke, but then they came too fast and her words became grunts, inarticulate noises of pain. Tears welled up in her eyes, and her ass flexed and danced. I wanted to make her let go, to break. I was angry at her for risking my career, and for making me desire her so much. I took that out on her, brought the crop down over and over, working her taut, red streaked buttocks, letting the tip snap into the tempting cleft between them. Her pussy was open now, her clit rigidly erect, peeking from beneath its protective hood, and I snapped the crop up against it. If she was so eager to be punished I was willing to make sure she got what she was looking for. The whipping seemed to go on forever, and finally I tore a word from her throat, choked out around her sobs.

"Please…"

"Please what?" *Snap*, I brought the crop down again.

"Please stop." *Snap*. "Sir." There was desperation in the word 'Sir'.

"Are you going to behave?" *Snap*.

"Yes sir." Her cunt had swollen more under the sting of the crop. The inner and outer lips opening to reveal the entrance to her vagina. Her hymen was intact. She was a virgin.

"Homework in on time?" *Snap*.

"Yes sir. Please sir."

The Teacher

"Well composed, well written, properly put together?" *Snap.*
"Yes sir. I'll be so good for you sir. Please stop."
"No more reading in class?" *Snap.*
"No sir, no sir, I'll be good, please stop, please please…"

I gave her one last stroke, drove it hard up between her legs so the shaft of the crop split her labia and the tip snapped against her clit. She screamed then, her cunt visibly pulsing under the impact as she shuddered hard, and it may be that she climaxed. I paused to breath. My cock was ready to burst and I wanted nothing more than to drive it up into that tight, wet, pink, and vulnerable hole. Instead I tossed the crop down and collapsed into my armchair. "We'll see on Monday, just how good you'll be."

"Yes sir. Thank you sir." She stayed in position, crying softly. Her ass was a solid mass of red welts. She'd have trouble sitting for a week. Her pussy was swollen and slick with her desire.

I tore my eyes from her display. "Get up. Go."

She stood up and turned to face me, her tear stained eyes begging for comfort. I just pointed to the door. I didn't want to build intimacy with her, I wanted her to understand that she was in too deep, that she couldn't handle what she thought she'd seen at the Club. She couldn't have been in my presence for more than five minutes, but it had seemed like forever. As soon as I hear the door close I hauled out my cock and started masturbating. It took me under a minute to finish, spurting huge globs of white hot sperm over my hand, my balls contracting so hard they hurt. The image of her tight, virgin cunt was burned into my brain. I was shaking at the end of it, and her vision filled my dreams that night.

Saturday dragged and Sunday dragged slower. She had me hooked though I didn't want to admit it. It wasn't just her body, it or her eager innocence. Part of it was her intelligence and maturity, so far in advance of her peer group, but there was more than that too, something deeper, something darker that showed in her eyes when they looked up into mine.

I understood when I thought about that, when I thought about her, how it was that she'd found herself at the Club. She was bored, not just with the advanced daycare centre we call high school but with her entire world, with the entire way of life in this bucolic little suburb, revolving as it did around shopping malls and high school football and the top ten shows on cable. A lot of girls in her situation discover drugs, use the high to lower their bar, submit themselves to the inexpert fumblings of half drunk jocks. Not her, she was too smart for that.

How many nights had she lain in her bed, surrounded by cute frilly things given to her by relatives who didn't understand the first thing about her, masturbating to visions of trial-by-ordeal? She would know how to defeat the parental controls on her computer and surf the darker corners of the internet.

She would know what was available, and she craved it and she had sensed in me that I had exactly that to offer, though with only the vaguest of idea of exactly what *that* was in reality. She had followed me and found it, and decided she wanted it, screwed her courage to the sticking point and found a way to get it.

The way to get it was to offer herself in trade, and I had found it an offer difficult to refuse. I was half tempted to call up her file and call her house, but that would be worse than stupid. She had what she wanted now and I wondered now what she thought of it. The demons set in. I had hoped to discourage her from her chosen path with a whipping too intense for her to take. She would be bruised, no question of that. What if her parents saw the welts, and asked her where they came from? What if she not only changed her mind but decided to tell on her own? Either way my career would end. Would it be worth it, to have a woman like her in my life? Would it be worth it, to avoid another Suzanne? My rational brain said not, but the decisions I had made disagreed with my rational brain. I had made my choices, and she had made hers, and there was nothing to do but wait.

Monday arrived like the change of the seasons, and the day seemed to unwind in slow motion while I felt every eye upon me, as if my colleagues could read the guilt written on my soul. It went on forever, until the last class of the day, until creative writing class. Julie came in and sat, at the front of the class, in the same pleated skirt she'd worn to my house, the same neat white blouse, her long dark hair was pulled back into a ponytail, alert and attentive and ready to learn. She was the perfect student, my perfect student, in every way. *In every way.* I went through the lesson in a haze, convinced every student could see our new-forged connection.

At the end of the class everyone handed in their papers, their weekend homework. She handed hers in last. It was entitled *Penitence*, six pages stapled together, laser printed, double spaced. It was the first assignment she'd handed in on time all year. There was a yellow sticky-note attached to the front page. 'Thank you for the extra attention in helping me complete my work. Julie.' I looked at it, looked at her. Her face was calm and composed. Behind me I heard the door click shut as the last student left.

I held up her assignment. "Will I be pleased with this?" I asked her.

"Yes, sir."

"Face the door." She did it. "Skirt up."

She flipped up her skirt to reveal her ass. She had thong underwear on this time, and though the welts had faded in most places, they had darkened in a few. I'd marked her, signed my name on her ass with my riding crop. She was mine, whether I wanted that or not, but I could not deny that I wanted it. A lot. Her ass was beautiful, firm and heart shaped, and the crotch of her thong was soaking wet.

"Skirt down." I said, resisting the urge to touch her offered pussy. I couldn't risk getting caught doing this, and yet there I was risking it. "Ten o'clock, my place."

"Yes sir." She went out and I waited until my erection had subsided enough to allow me to walk in public. It would be harder for her to get out on a school night than on a Friday. I didn't want it to end now, I just needed it to.

Another endless night of waiting. I read her story, *Penitence*. It told of a Catholic girl in confessional, atoning for her sins with oral sex offered through a hole in the confessional screen. "Bless me Father, for I have sinned," it began, and before the end she receives her blessing, a baptism sprayed on her face from her Father's guiding staff. It was dark and explicit, completely inappropriate, and it was stunningly good.

At ten the door chimed. At three minutes past she was bent over my desk again, hands grabbing the far side, legs spread wide, her tight, no-longer virgin cunt clamped around my cock as she screamed out her orgasm. I fucked her forever, my hands squeezing her bruised ass cheeks hard, making her beg for it, making her feel it, making her come over and over, until her contractions became painful, until she begged me to stop. I didn't stop, I kept fucking her, my cock like a steel bar, over and over, on and on.

When at last I unloaded my balls into her I nearly passed out. I meant to send her home promptly, mindful of parental curfews, but she told me her parents were away. I could have her as much as I wanted. Later that night she crawled for me. She kissed my boots, licked them, worshipped them. She knelt for me and sucked me, exactly as in her story, and then I fucked her again, and again, and again.

It was not lovemaking, it was sex, raw and violent, passions unbridled. It was conquest and submission, each of us playing our half of the duet. But when it was over, when I had fucked her and whipped her and tied her and pumped her so full of sperm that my balls ached, wrung absolutely dry, when we were both so drained neither one of us could stand, then the inevitable emotions set in. I lay on my bed, sweaty and sated, exhausted and trembling and she put the tangled mop of her hair on my chest and cuddled close and said "Thank you, Sir," with a purr of contentment, and I held her until it was far too late, and she finally went home just in time to beat the dawn.

She came in her own car I learned. Her parents had bought it for her birthday. It was the same one she had taken into the city, to the Club, to follow an instinct she was only now beginning to understand. I fell asleep when she left, exhausted and with just three hours before the alarm was due to wake me. *Alea iacta est.* The die was cast, the Rubicon left far behind. Julie and I would play this out, as far as it would go.

I learned over the next month just how far that might be. There was nothing she would not do. My memory of that time is full of images flash frozen in my brain with sexual intensity, Julie kneeling to suck my cock, Julie kneeling with her tongue extended and covered in sperm, waiting for permission to swallow. Julie's face in the mirror, contorted in mingled pleasure and pain as I came hard up her tight little ass. Julie with her nose in the corner, skirt up to expose a fresh set of welts, Julie with nipple clamps, with cunt clamps, Julie gagged, Julie trussed, Julie crawling, Julie begging for punishment, for orgasm, for me to cum on her and in her. Julie used and abused and degraded every way I could think of to do it. She lapped it all up, and then demanded more.

    I changed her arrival time to seven to give me more time to take her, and my world became Julie. Her parents spent a lot of time away, which explained her ease in staying out late. That was purely lucky for me because by then I didn't care about getting caught. Psychoanalysis might hint that the reason she came to me, the reason she needed what I offered, was due to her parent's emotional absence, but my role in her life was not to provide analysis but catharsis. And Julie provided me with what I needed in return, provided it in full measure. She was my drug, addictive and compelling, lithe limbed and pliant, soaking up everything I could give her. And all the time her schoolwork got better and better, she kept her side of the bargain. I checked her file after midterm exams, and her marks were all either A or A+. The other teachers in the staffroom remarked on the change in her attitude, little guessing what was bringing it about. Her writing changed too, from dark themes to light, from despair to hope. I've seen that change before, in the women who respond to what it is I offer. I've never seen it so dramatically as in Julie.

    I took risks, too many risks. I trained her to spread her legs on a signal in class, so I could see her wet cunt while her classmates paid attention to what I'd put on the board. I trained her to climax on command, and then gave her that command while she had her legs spread in class. I fucked her in the classroom after school with the door locked and her wrists cuffed behind her back. I fucked her at lunch with a ring gag in her mouth. She came to school with rope marks burned red into her wrists, and her ass was always marked and sore. I don't know how she dealt with that in the locker room or at home. I don't know what she told her friends about where she went each night. I was jeopardizing my career and I didn't even care. My prep-work went on autopilot because she occupied all my time every night she could get free, and all my thoughts on the nights she couldn't. What mattered was Julie, nothing else.

    On the day after Thanksgiving she spent the evening kneeling beneath my desk with her face in my lap, her lips wrapped around my cock, sucking eagerly while I read her Act V from Shakespeare's Macbeth. It had become our standard instructional position. The reading was next week's homework assignment. It was routine now for her to kneel there, servicing my shaft as I read to her. The ritual had become comforting in its familiarity, and yet I could

The Teacher

not repress a shudder that was more than sexual as Macbeth's wife cried "Out, out, damned spot," as she scrubbed in vain to cleanse her blood-stained hands. I was stained with the blood of Julie's virginity as surely as Lady Macbeth was stained with the blood of Banquo's life.

My crime was there for all to see, written in her sundered hymen, written in the welts that never quite had time to fade from her ass before I gave her more. I read the passage again and realized that I had to end it. It was not just my career but my soul I'd put at risk. No matter how right it felt, it was still wrong, and I had to stop this while I still had the chance. I put the book down and looked down at her, her big eyes wide and worshipful as they looked up at me, her full red lips working my hard cock just the way I'd taught her.

She slid herself back, to the point where her lips were just grazing the head of my cock. "Please come on my face, sir," she pleaded. "Please make me be your dirty little whore."

Desire hit me like a tidal wave, over-riding every fear, every doubt. I grabbed her hair, thrust my cock back in, seeking the back of the throat with the swollen head. It was hard for her to take it that deep but she did it. She did everything, that's the way she was, and she thrived on being made to do it. She loved the thick rigid shaft forcing her jaw wide, the soft, firm texture of the head, the salty, slippery precum dripping on her tongue.

It occurred to me that I hadn't been to the Club since the first night she'd come to me. She made them all pale in comparison, Lize and the rest. I looked again into her eyes, held her head in my hands as my cock stiffened rigid, getting ready to spurt. She knew what was coming, she knew my responses by now. Her eyes widened, her expression totally accepting, and almost without warning my orgasm hit, my balls contracting, emptying spurt after spurt of sperm down her eager sucking throat. My juice her mouth until it ran down her chin, and dripped down to glaze her firm, full tits.

She sighed in satisfaction, her eyes sliding closed as she swallowed. She was allowed to swallow automatically when I read to her, and she never failed to tremble in pleasure at the privilege, her cunt contracting in gentle orgasm without so much as touching her clit. I leaned back, reclining to allow her to suckle my softening cock clean. And I knew then that I couldn't stop. I truly was addicted to her, eager little minx that she was, even as she was addicted to me. I couldn't give her up, come what may, and I hated myself for my weakness, even as I took strength from my conquest of her cunt.

And then it was December, report card time. With it came Parent's Day, and with Parent's Day came Julie's father. Her mother was away at some social function, and he, like his daughter, waited until the end of the evening, waited at the back of the line so he could talk to me alone. He was older than I'd expected, grey haired and well dressed, with an air of authority. He was a lawyer, Julie had told me, a partner at a well established firm, and his handshake was solid. He obviously took advantage of the corporate fitness plan.

"Good evening," he said, as I locked the door behind us and he walked me out to my car. "I want to thank you for taking the time to do extra work with Julie. My wife and I can't believe the change in her."

"She's a talented girl," I replied, and he couldn't have understood all the ways in which I meant it.

"She's worried us for a long time. She hasn't seemed to care much about her future."

"Julie isn't the average student. She needs a different approach." He little knew how different that approach was.

"Maybe so, but you're the only one who's taken the time to give it to her."

"She's a lot smarter than her peer group. Quite frankly she's a lot smarter than a lot of my colleagues. That can be more of a burden than a blessing."

"Not smarter than you, eh?" He gave me a nudge and a smile, inviting me into the old boy's club for a moment.

I shook my head. "No, she's smarter than me I think." *Smart enough to seduce me into our dangerous little game.* "I've just managed to gain some rapport with her, win her respect enough that she'll put in effort."

He nodded ruefully. "I wish I could do that."

"It's different," I said, "You're her father. She's trying to grow up and make her own way."

"I know." He looked away, and I saw him wish for the days when his little girl was really still his little girl, jumping up into daddy's big strong arms for a hug, laughing in delight at a magic trick or a new kitten, begging for another bedtime story or an extra cookie when Mom wasn't looking. I couldn't tell him just how much his daughter had grown up in the last few months, I couldn't tell him how very little of his little girl was left. I couldn't tell him how I had won her respect, in a way that would be forever closed to him. I certainly couldn't tell him that she was waiting for me that very moment, having let herself in to my house with her key, that she was waiting, bent over my desk with her long legs spread and her skirt up ready to be whipped or fucked at my whim. I might perhaps have told him that she had missed him growing up, that he shouldn't have spent so many late nights at the firm, that he should have given her fewer things and more time, that the one thing she craved more than anything was Daddy's love and approval. I couldn't tell him that his absence was ultimately what had brought her to me.

If she were younger I could have told him those things and perhaps they would have made a difference, but she was no longer a girl, she was a woman, and now it was too late. I shook his hand and felt guilty. *Bless me Father, for I have sinned.* I have despoiled your daughter, I have ruined her for the sharp, clean-cut, up-and-coming law/medicine/MBA student you're hoping she'll meet in university. No fine young man will suffice to slake her thirst now that I've had my hands on her, now that I've dirtied her with my desire. She will excel, she will succeed at everything you dream for her, and you will be proud of her, but you will never feel that connection you're only now realizing you've lost. And you will never know the moment when she chooses someone just like dear old Dad.

    I left him there, got into my car and drove home. She was on time and in position and my cock was rigid before I could get my belt undone. I swung hard once, just to hear the crack of leather on flesh and to see her jump and hear her moan, and then I was fucking her, driving my stiff shaft up into her tight receptive body and I forgot it all, my career, her father, everything. The only thing that mattered was my eager student, my star pupil, my woman, my Julie. I thrust harder, feeling my orgasm build, my balls clenching tight and contracting as I roared out my triumph and emptied myself into her one more time. My knees went weak and I pulled her to the floor, to lie there still tangled with her, still inside her. And in that moment I found myself at peace.

Part Five

And you, honey. Are you Julie, were you Julie? Were you too smart for your peer group in school, too smart for the adults in your world? Was it a teacher you pined after, some strong, smart, tall, dark, handsome, older man? Or did that come later, with a prof in university? I know you're a reader, because books like this don't find their way into the hands of women who spend their lives in front of the television. Did you escape into books, rebel like Julie did? Or were you a dutiful student like Suzanne, making the grade for a gold star and the right to be left alone by parents and teachers alike? And what books did you read on your own time? What thought first made you wet between the legs? Julie read *this* book, did you catch that? She read her own story here, just as you're reading yours.

Oh yes, I know your story, it's written in your secret thoughts, the fantasies that bubble beneath the surface of your nice-girl veneer. How many boyfriends have you toyed with, played with and ultimately thrown away because they couldn't give you that? How many times have you tried to ask for it and been misunderstood? People don't understand this kind of interaction, this little dynamic you and I are playing out here. They think it's about what they see, they think it's about leather and latex, pain and pleasure, restraint and discipline. They don't understand that it's about the mind.

But it is *all* about the mind, about that secret place you hide deep inside, everything else is just a tool to open that inner door. *I* am all about the mind and when I say *I want you* what I want is your mind, if only because I know your body will follow. So come through the door once more, honey, come through the door and into my classroom because it's time for me to instruct you, to induct you. It's time to teach you what happens to good girls and bad girls in my world. It's time for you to learn exactly how to present yourself to present your oral report.

Read between the lines honey, I know you're clever enough to see the message written there. I have faith in your ability, or at least faith that you'll do what I want when the alternative is the riding crop applied to your ripe, swollen, well spread cunt. Did you feel the sting when Julie took it on the crotch? Imagine it, feel it now, that sharp-sweet *snap* that strikes to your core and reminds you so very effectively of the purpose of our journey. We're going to play our own little game of teacher-and-student now, honey. You get to be the student, and as I'm sure you're well aware the schoolroom game is all about marks, marks on paper and marks on your ass. So park your hot little ass down at your desk and I'll give you this week's assignment, homework in essay form.

Question One: It is generally considered immoral for a teacher to carry on a sexual relationship with a student, and the teacher in this story struggles with this. What influence did Julie's desire for him have on his decision? What influence does his own desire have? What does he get out of the relationship? What does she get out of it? What do you think will happen? Twenty five marks.

Question Two: Compare and contrast your own sexual development with that of Julie. Use explicit reference to your own early sexual fantasies of domination by a man of intelligence and authority. Twenty five marks.

Question Three: The story is written entirely from the teacher's point of view. Imagine you are Julie. How did you feel when you first knelt and asked for training? How did you feel when your teacher said yes? How did you feel when you bent over his desk to be whipped for the first time? How did you feel when he came in your cunt? In your mouth? In your ass? Twenty five marks.

Question Four: You're a dirty little slut and I've just caught you reading this book with wet panties when you should be doing your homework. How should you be punished? Be detailed, explicit and imaginative. Twenty five marks.

The assignment is due one week from today.

There it is honey, your homework. I just know that you're going to get all one hundred marks on it. I know because every mark you don't get with your writing is going to be burned into your ass. Are you surprised at this little turn of events, honey? I bet you thought you'd spend all your time with me reading and none at all writing, but that's not the way it works. This little game requires class participation. So let me be very clear about the participation I expect, and that is for you to have your assignment done, complete, spelling checked and grammar correct, between three and five hundred words per question with the title underlined, in the centre, at the top. You will have your name in the upper right and Creative Writing 101 in the upper left. It will be neatly handwritten, in black ink, double spaced on white bond notebook paper with one inch margins. I expect nothing but perfection from you honey, so you'd better not let me down.

Have you got that clear in your mind? Good girl. And wouldn't you rather be having fun diddling your hot little pussy to my compelling and erotic prose than doing homework? You didn't even get to orgasm last time and this time you're doing homework. And yes, honey, I know just how much your clit is throbbing right now, I know just how badly you need release, need to have it stroked and rubbed with that ready, steady rhythm until your world explodes. I know how much you want to give that to me, even more than you want to give it to yourself. But this is part of the process honey, this is what makes our journey real and so you're going to focus your mind on your task right now, and I am just going to have to wait for the glory of your orgasm no matter how much I want it. Discipline starts with self-discipline. And speaking of self-discipline, you're not allowed to climax until you're done.

So say, "Yes," honey. Say, "Yes," the way you do for me.

"Yes, sir. I'll be a good girl and get my homework done on time." Say it.

"Yes Sir, I'll be disciplined." Say it.

"Yes Sir, please discipline me." Feel it. Feel the way Julie felt, asking for it, needing it, responding to it, craving it, demanding it and lost in it. Feel yourself being directed in the direction you need to go, corrected by this strong, smart, tall, dark, handsome man who makes your knees so weak you have no choice but to kneel for him.

And do you know what, honey? I believe in hands-on education. I believe people learn best through doing, so now that we're training you, teaching you, I think we can make this a very instructive experience. So we know that you're now going to be spending a certain number of hours at a desk, and what we're going to do to further the cause of classroom participation is to make sure you are very thoroughly penetrated while you do it. So I don't care if you use a carrot or a vibrator and I don't care if it goes in your mouth or your ass or your cunt, but the entire time you're writing you're going to be penetrated because that's your role here, to receive cock as you receive knowledge, to be instructed and inseminated at the very same time.

That hard penetrating shaft is going to be there to be my cock for you and you're going to receive it while you receive instruction. You're going to take it just like Julie did, sucking away while she listened to her Shakespeare lesson. It's going to take you several hours at least, hours with your lips wrapped around my phallic stand-in, hours with your tight stretched anus violated, hours with your pussy full and juicing. So don't cheat me honey, don't cheat yourself. You're going to do this assignment first and you're not going to read more of this book until you're finished. That would spoil the sequence honey, that would spoil the adventure that I've built here for you, so don't do it, be a good girl for me. Homework first and reward later for good behaviour by good girls, and yes, honey, I promise it will be a very good reward.

So say, "Yes," honey.

"Yes sir, I'll do my homework first. Yes sir, I'll have it in on time."

It makes you wet to say that doesn't it? Being put in this position goes straight to your cunt, whether you like it or not. You're so turned on you could scream, couldn't you honey? You're rocking your hips again, you feel that need to arch your back, spread your legs, present your cunt and just have me slam-fuck you until the orgasm gets ripped right out of your body. You want more

Part Five

but I'll tell you something, honey. You've undertaken to get your homework done. You're not going to start reading this again until your homework *is* done, so that desire will give you incentive to do it quickly. Say, "Yes, sir," one last time honey, and put the book down. I'm looking forward to reading what you're about to write.

Cage Girl

Society is a cage, and a cruel one. Its bars are made of propriety, its lock with expectation. Society's cage was made for me by others but, ultimately, I'm the one who put myself in it. The problem is, I've forgotten how to let myself out. My cage, the one I'm in right now, is simpler. It has metal bars and a wooden floor and roof. Unlike society's cage, I built it. I bought the wood and metal, cut it to fit, sanded and polished, stained and screwed, but I don't put myself in it. You have to understand that. I am a competent woman, educated, ambitious, professional, independent. At work I'm well respected, at home I can do my own carpentry and fix my own car. Restraint, constraint is the one thing I can't do for myself. *He* does that for me, and in caging me here he frees me from society's cage.

He doesn't do it for that reason, he does it to remind me of my place as his possession, but the cage is more than that. In a very real way it *is* my place. I find my centre there, at peace, because there is nothing I can do until he decides to let me out. Sometimes I'm hooded in there, ears plugged, eyes covered, mouth gagged. Sometimes I'm bound in a position so strict that the cage itself becomes unnecessary except as an attractive display case for my body. At times like those I can feel myself collapsing into myself, almost as if the woman I am in the daytime is dissolving away, her emotions, her needs, her moods, her temper washed clean, with nothing left behind.

I can feel myself regress from that woman, the one with impeccable style and outstanding taste, the calm, in-control leader, the one who saves a dozen lives a day. I can feel myself slip away as my lack of control is made so abundantly clear. None of what I am matters in my cage, not my achievements, not my discomfort, not even my name. All that counts is the fact of my physical existence, and the fact that I am *his*. I'm kept caged for hours sometimes, curled up naked, unable to stretch out or sit up. It's anything but comfortable being in there and I'm sore and stiff when I come out. And yet I miss my cage when I'm out of it too long. It is far less cruel than society's.

This isn't to say that my cage is easy. When I'm first put in, it can be very hard. I become like an adolescent, moody and defiant. I struggle against the bonds, fight against them, scream into the gag. I am angry and demanding and, because I am who I am, I expect to get my way, to have my demands met, even though, with the calmer, more rational part of my mind, I know they won't be. This is the only place in my life where I don't get my way, and sometimes it takes me awhile to remind myself of that fact.

And yet after a time I grow tired, and the struggles diminish. The bonds envelope me, hold me, protect me from the damage I might inflict on myself or anyone near. They defend me from the guilt of a lost temper, they hold me back from my own excess. I regress more then, become in my heart a young child, quiet and obedient. I accept my position, as humiliating as it may be. And then, slowly, slowly, even the child subsides and I return to the womb, to drift in warm darkness with nothing but the steady beat of my own pulse in my ears. I am free in that place, as I am free no-where else in my life.

I have learned to be careful with whom I share this secret. Friends have looked at me strangely, awkwardly changed the topic when I stray too near to the workings of my private life. Before I met *him* I had suggested to lovers that perhaps we experiment with rope, with blindfolds and perhaps, just maybe, with more. Too many times I was repulsed, told I was sick, that I needed psychiatric help. For too long I believed there was something deeply wrong with me. I was locked in society's cage, while I yearned for my own.

I have always driven myself harder, held myself to a higher standard than anyone else. I have always fought to be on top, in school, in business, in relationships, and I always, always win. And yet, deep down, I have always had the desire to give that up, yearned to meet someone strong enough to put me in my place and to keep me there, to take me off my pedestal - no, to knock me off my pedestal, and put me at their feet. It could have been a man, it could have been a woman, it didn't matter. In the event it was a man, and he changed my life.

I spend at least an hour a day in the cage, sometimes more. Sometimes when I'm hooded and trussed and gagged in there he slides a dildo into my pussy, to remind me of exactly what my role is. It's a simple role. I service his cock. In this cage I am not called by my name, not by the honorific title I earned in years of hard work in school. In this cage I am just *cunt*. That's a simple anatomical underlining of the reality that underpins our relationship. The dildo will stretch me wide, probe humiliatingly deep and I am powerless to stop it. More importantly, I am powerless to stop my body's response to his casual control.

The dildo never finds resistance, it always finds me slick and wet and swollen, eager for any form of touch from him. I'm *his* cunt, his ready, willing, eager cunt, and yes it's humiliating to say that about myself. He's trained me to be his cunt, to be always open and wet for him. I struggle with that sometimes, just as I struggle against the bonds in the cage. I struggle because it is my instinct to struggle, though I neither expect nor even want to win. Like the bonds, I know I can't break away from the fundamental reality. I. Am. His.

Cunt. I couldn't imagine being that way for anyone else. I couldn't imagine being any other way with him.

Sometimes he takes me out, still trussed, and fucks me until he's done with me, and then puts me back in, now sweaty and dripping with his sperm. Sometimes he'll have a ring gag in my mouth and use my mouth through it, spraying his juices on my face and tongue. Sometimes he ass-fucks me, driving his shaft up between my offered buttocks while I hang suspended between pleasure and pain. When he takes me his cock becomes something more than simple flesh and blood. It becomes the living embodiment of his authority, and my various sexual openings become the portals through which his authority is injected into me. Every time he fucks me my submission is reinforced. Every time he fucks me I become more and more his cunt.

Cunt.

At this point in our relationship he doesn't need the cage, doesn't need the hood, doesn't need the whip or any other device. All it takes is a glance, a gesture for him to put me into the appropriate position of receptiveness, kneeling with my mouth open, down on all fours with my ass in the air, flat on my back in the horizontal splits. All those accessories are for me now, to allow me to feel properly confined, to feel safely restrained, to feel my inner demons channeled into constructive directions.

Accordingly I have to beg for them. I have to crawl to him with the cuffs and the hood in my teeth. I have to wait for him on all fours with the riding crop held in the cleft of my ass and a note explaining in detail why I need to be punished. Sometimes the reason is real, a moment of lost temper, or neglect of some detail at work or at home. More often now the reason is simply because I need it, need deep down to have my demons scourged out, need to offer up my pain to him, need to show him how much I am *his*. The simple truth is I need to be humiliated in order to escape from myself. I need to be stripped and bared and transformed into *cunt*.

Part of that transformation has been his mastery of my orgasms. Before him I came easily on my own through masturbation and almost never with a partner. He has trained me now to orgasm at his command, and only at his command. No matter what I do, however much I rub my clit with my time honoured technique, I can't come by myself, though he can make me do it with a word, over and over again if he wants to, until my pussy is sore and aching from clenching, until the experience is no longer pleasurable but painful, until I am limp and exhausted and begging for him to stop as eagerly as I begged for him to start. It's something I wouldn't have thought possible before I met him, and now it's an everyday part of my reality.

When I had control of my own orgasms, sex was something I rarely thought about. Now sex, specifically the image of his cock imposing its will on me, never leaves my mind. As a result I spend my days in a state of barely contained sexual frustration. Everything I see, everything I touch seems to remind me of his cock. I have to pack extra underwear with my lunch to work, in the certain knowledge I will have soaked through several pairs of it before the day is done, as my obsession with him seizes my thoughts. Sexual release has become one more thing I have to grovel for, and so I am highly motivated to be a very good cunt for him.

He has trained me so I need it often. The one time I am always allowed to come is when he has shot his sperm into me, and that makes me eager to present my sex openings for his use. He has conditioned me to crave his cock, to be a slave, quite literally, to his cock. I'm lucky that he knows how to do that with consummate skill, lucky enough that he chooses to invest that skill in me. You may wonder why any sane woman would choose to submit herself to such treatment, let alone consider herself lucky to be subjected to it. This simple fact is that I do not choose to do this, any more than you can choose to breathe. I need it, and I have long since passed the point of wondering if my need is right or wrong. It simply is.

And so I lie in here, encased in leather, joints aching from the tight restraints he has put me in, hooded, ears plugged, mouth held open by the ring gag. My wrists are cuffed behind my back, my ankles cuffed to my wrists. My feet are encased in high heeled leather boots, my hands in monogloves that deny me the use of my fingers. A tight corset cinches my waist, accentuating my tits and ass beneath the smooth leather, and the only part of my body exposed to the outside air is my spread, swollen, dripping cunt.

I strain to hear any noise that might indicate he has come to touch me. Time contracts and expands and I lose all orientation, all sense of the outside world. I become lost in my own thoughts and I regress, the cares of the world washed away. My awareness focuses on my cunt and its desire to be put to its rightful use. My arousal grows, my stiff clit aching for stimulation, and I try to hump it against the cage floor, although I know my restraints won't allow me to. Time passes and eventually I *become* my cunt, my entire body sensitized to the point where it is merely an extension of my vagina.

And then I feel it, the slight vibration that means the cage door has been opened. Hands pull me backwards, and then his cock enters me, fully, deeply, with no preparation, stretching me to the point of pain. I gasp and moan, the discomfort of my position transformed in an instant to arousal, and then he is fucking me the way I need so much to be fucked, and I want to beg him to come in me, to use me, to make *cunt* into *his* cunt. His cock is steel hard, its thick, heavy head pounding remorselessly against my cervix, and I want to beg him to come inside me, so deep inside me, but I can't, because the cruel ring gag renders my aching mouth incapable of speech, incapable of anything but accepting his cock, should he choose to use me that way too.

The Secret Journey

But right now he's using my cunt, using me as his cunt, and it is exactly what I need and it goes on and on until I can't think, can't even remember my own name and all I can feel is my stretched, fucked pussy as he slams into me over and over and over again. I can do nothing but take it, and I want nothing more than to be made to take it. And then his hands tighten on my ass, his cock stiffens, swells even more as his final thrust impales me to the very centre of my being. I hear him grunting, moaning, roaring. I feel his balls, rammed hard against my ass as they are, pulsing powerfully as he pumps his rich, thick seed into my open, receptive hole.

I come. The world goes black. Later he will let me out. Tomorrow I will go to work and again be called by name, be called by my honorific title. I will have the respect of my colleagues, their admiration, even their envy. Tomorrow I will be brilliant and in control. That's tomorrow. Right now I am cunt, and he has completed me.

Part Six

Welcome back, honey. Did you like cunt's story? Did it make you wet, did you envy her the clear simplicity of her relationship? It doesn't matter, because the more important question is, is your homework done?

Visualize the classroom door, feel yourself come through it, feel it close behind you. Visualize the classroom, the empty desks, the clean-slate chalkboard. See the teacher's desk, my desk, the desk over which you'll be bent for your corrections. The door is closed behind you and it's just you and me for our after-school lessons. Feel me there with you, watching you, and be on your attentive, classroom best behaviour. Remember that little assignment, from part five? Did you take it seriously, or did you just skip ahead because you thought you could get away with it. Is it done? Is it done well? Am I going to be pleased with it? Your heart thumps at that, knowing that you're going to be tested soon. Is it because you haven't done it? It's possible you're just reading ahead because you haven't yet learned that this is more than just a book.

You've got one last chance now, the final reprieve before the bell rings. I want your homework paper in hand when you turn the page, honey. Your paper, and a red pen, and the instrument of your correction. That last one is key. It doesn't matter what it is, a wooden spoon or a riding crop or a hairbrush, just so long its application will leave a lasting impression, on your ass and on your mind. That made your heart skip a beat, didn't it honey? You see where this is going now, don't you? And you are going to be staring at this page wondering if you're going to go through with it. Only you *are* going to go through with it honey, because you don't want to break the spell. You're well into the journey now, the door is closed behind you, and you don't want it to stop, you want to feel the way I make you feel. You want it more than anything, you want it so bad you're going to be dreaming about it every night for weeks after I finally give it to you. You're going to be dreaming naughty, bad girl dreams that wet the sheets and wake you up hot and needy.

So no, honey, you don't want to break the spell, and that means you're going to go ahead, go get it, that hard tool that's going to soften you up, that's going to correct your ass and attitude, as we correct your homework. Get it, and your paper, and your red pen. Go and get what you need. Stop reading and get it. Right now.

Part Six

And now you're back, and you're holding your own fate in your hands, paper in one hand, punishment in the other. Put the paper down, because before we begin we're going to test out your punishment. Heft it, swish it, feel it, try it out, honey. Imagine how it's going to feel on your ass if your homework isn't up to standard. Feel the tight little knot of anticipation in your belly. You're longing to try it out, just to feel it, just to have some understanding of the experience you're about to have. So go ahead, honey, smack your ass with it. Do it hard, don't be shy, it's just you and me here. Smack it hard enough to feel it, listen to the impact, listen to the crack, feel the heat. Do it again honey, turn the other cheek for me, do it hard, make it sting. And if it didn't sting enough, if you don't think I'd be satisfied with the instensity of that *smack*, do it again, both cheeks. Do it until you do it right, until it's hard enough to make you want to be a good girl for me.

Oh yes, honey, we want you to be a good girl, don't we? And now we know how to motivate you towards good behaviour. So now it's time to mark your paper, a little academic exercise that you're going to do naked. That's right, honey, strip for me, if you're not stripped already, but leave the panties on, I like a girl in panties. Remember Julie's thong? Remember the way it split her welted ass when she was put on display? Remember how her crotch was soaked? Yeah, you can feel your own crotch getting slippery, I know you can. Put a finger down and check, and put it back up to your lips and taste yourself. Bad, bad, girl. We'll deal with that wetness later, but right now we're going to see how your grades measure up.

So let's turn to your paper now honey, get your homework and get your red pen and we're going to evaluate it. Every point lost is a red mark, and every red mark on the page is going to wind up as a red mark on your ass. Are you ready honey? Check for your name in the upper right, check for the title at the top, in the centre. It should be a title that makes sense, like "Assignment One - The Teacher".

Check for Homeroom 4A in the upper left. Evaluate the handwriting, is it neat, is it clear and legible? Is it worthy of you? Red mark if the name's not there, red mark if the title isn't right, red mark if the homeroom isn't there, red mark if the handwriting isn't perfect, lose another point if it's sloppy, lose another if it's actually messy, lose another if the title isn't underlined. Five red marks if it isn't handwritten, if you cheated and used a printer. I expect my instructions to be carried out, honey, exactly as I give them. Check the margins. Are they even? If not, red mark. Are they an inch exactly? If not, red mark.

Now question one, honey, remember that? You need to explain the effect of Julie's desire on her teacher, and that of his own desire. You have to predict what's going to happen with them, and discuss the dynamic of their relationship. So sit up straight in your chair and take your paper and read it aloud with red pen in hand. Read it in a clear voice, and as you read it evaluate

The Secret Journey

it, listen to the words, the phrasing, the sentence structure. And every time you come to an error, grammar or spelling, that's a red mark. Every time the phrasing is awkward or the point is unclear, red mark. Be strict, honey, as strict as I would be. Stop reading this now, and read your work aloud.

Part Six

Now that you're finished, ask yourself if you were convincing. Ask yourself if you expressed yourself as well as you possibly could have. Ask yourself if this work is up to the standard that I would expect from you, that you would expect from yourself. Red marks every time you don't get a good answer to those questions, honey, as many red marks as there needs to be. Don't be easy on yourself honey, the idea isn't to cheat and cut corners, the idea is to learn and to learn we need to be honest here. Right now we're setting the standard, and you have high standards, because that's who you are, that's why you're here. And ask yourself if your reading voice was clear and articulate. Red mark if it wasn't. Finish your marking, and then turn the page.

Part Six

Question two, honey. Tell me about your sexual development, your sexual fantasies of domination by a man of intelligence and authority. Read them out loud, too. You know the standard now. We're not here to judge your fantasies, anything you dream is absolutely fine, but that red pen is going to move for spelling, for grammar, for every other technical detail that's less than perfect for me. Don't be afraid to express yourself honey, and don't be afraid to mark yourself. And tell me did writing your thoughts down bring a blush to your cheeks? Did writing your thoughts down bring them one step closer to real? Of course it did, and you know the real reason behind this question, don't you, honey? You know that I want to know what buttons to push in your mind. And because you know the purpose of this question, that's ten red marks if you evaded it, if you weren't absolutely honest about the darkest corners of your desire. Intellectual dishonesty is the worst academic sin, and I won't have it in my class.

And speaking of buttons, I bet your hot little button is hard right now, and I bet your panties are well on their way to soaking wet. Is it your own fantasies that are doing that to you honey, or is it all the red marks on your paper, and the knowledge that very, very soon now they're going to be on your ass? You're looking forward to that, I know you are. Not so much the hot, sharp smack but the fact that you'll be getting it from me, that I'll be providing you with exactly what you need, whether you want it or not. And red mark if I just caught you slouching in your chair. Back straight, honey. Posture is important. Read your work aloud, and grade it like before, and turn the page when you're done.

Part Six

    Question three, honey. How do you feel about kneeling and asking to be trained? How do you feel bent over the desk to be whipped? How do you feel being fucked with your ass all sore and welted and red and swollen? How do you feel about being fucked like that, being required to suck my cock like that, taking it up the ass like that? And what do you get from this relationship? Read it aloud honey, and make your red marks just like you're supposed to. Stop reading this now, and read your work aloud.

Part Six

Last question, honey, how should dirty little sluts like you be punished? Tell me in detail honey. Tell me what needs to be done so I can do it to you. You need to be kept in line, I know that much. You need to be taught how to respect the cock. Read it loud and proud honey, and evaluate it just like the other three questions. Red marks for grammar, for spelling, for writing and margins. Red marks when you aren't up to the required level of articulate presentation. And ten red marks if you skated the question, made the punishment any lighter than the full measure that you need. I need you open, honey, I won't have anything less. Stop reading this now, and read your work aloud.

Part Six

And now, honey, we're going to add up all those red marks. Are you sitting up straight right now, honey? Three red marks if I caught you slouching again. Just because you're getting all wet and squirmy is no reason to relax the requirements. And let's do that, let's check how wet you are, naughty, dirty girl. Have you soaked right through your panties, made a mess on the schoolroom chair? Put your hand down there and check, bad girl, that's a red mark if your cunt is wet, another if your panties are, and five if you've made your chair sticky. Is your clit stiff? Check it, honey, red mark if it is. Are you a hot little cocksucking bitch? We already know you are honey, we proved that back in part three. Five red marks for being such a bad, bad girl.

So count them up honey, count up all the red marks so we can bring you right up to perfect. And just in case you've skipped ahead honey, just in case you're reading this without your homework done, it's twenty five red marks for every question you didn't do, plus the ones for slouching, for being a bad girl, for being a hot little cocksucking bitch, and twenty five extra for deliberately avoiding the work. So I hope you did make an effort honey, I hope you didn't skip your assignment, because otherwise you're going to have a lot of trouble sitting this week. Count them up now, and then turn the page.

Part Six

    Good girl, my bad girl. How many red marks did you earn? The number is important, because now your backside is going to be presented and punished honey. Every red mark on your page is going to be made up on your ass, so bend yourself over the desk or the table or the dresser or whatever it is you have to be bent over. Get your back arched, get your ass up and out and yes, of course, get your legs apart, wide, wide apart. This book in one hand, and your instrument of correction in the other. Get in position, honey. We're going to make you a very good girl indeed.

Part Six

First things first, bad girl. I'm going to show you how to do it like I do it. The most important thing is the way you count them, and the way you count them is this. The spanks come down, hard and sharp and one stroke at a time, and afterward you say, "One, sir. Thank you for making me be a good girl, sir. Please may I have another?" Then another spank and, "Two, sir. Thank you for making me be a good girl, sir. Please may I have another?" Then another and. "Three, sir, thank you for making me be a good girl, sir. Please may I have another?" You're going to say that for each spank, unless the spank isn't quite hard enough, and then you'll say. "Please sir, I need it harder, may I have that one again?" And the way you know it's hard enough is if you hear a definite, hard smack on impact, and it makes you jump and gasp and sends lightning bolts through your body. The way you know it's hard enough is that you'll be thinking – *Please I can't take it, that's too hard.* Anything less than that doesn't count. "Please sir, I need it harder, may I have that one again?"

How wet are you now, naughty girl, bent over like this awaiting your punishment? Are you eager for it or reluctant? Curious? Scared? Both at once, and more than that, you're aroused. Your heart is beating fast and your belly is tight and yes, your nipples are starting to stiffen. Your breathing is coming faster and your lips are dry and so part them honey, lick them. And now we'll begin.

First spank. *Now!*

"One sir. Thank you for making me a good girl, sir. Please may I have another?"

Second spank. *Now!*

"Two sir. Thank you for making me a good girl, sir. Please may I have another?"

And that's the way it's going to work, honey. Just keep going, spank after spank, thank me for each and ask for the next until every last one has been driven home, until every last red mark has been paid for in full. Rhythmic and steady, that's the way it has to be. Smack, smack, smack.

Yes honey, I know it hurts. And you know you need it to hurt. We both know you need this, you know you have been needing this for a long time. Is it bringing tears to your eyes, honey? Are you going to have trouble sitting tomorrow? If not you aren't doing it hard enough. So do it harder, honey. You're going to be doing it as hard as I would, and that's very hard indeed, hard enough to turn your luscious ass cheeks red, hard enough to make you squirm and dance and gasp and cry.

Harder, honey. That's the way. Show me how much you want to be a good girl. Let me strip away the badness, let me scourge your soul clean. Just take it honey, just accept it. Show me what a good girl you can be for me. It's just about you and me honey, and you should understand that I have your best interests at heart here. This is done because I want nothing but the best for you, nothing but the best from you. You do understand that, don't you, honey? What you might not understand is that this is hard for me too. I don't like to have to do this, but we both know it has to be done.

Harder, honey. How many are you up to now? Finish them off, rhythmic and steady, no drop in intensity, no change in cadence. Do it, honey, do it hard, and if you aren't pleased with your own response, if you don't feel I'd be pleased with the intensity, or with the way you hold your posture or the clarity of your voice when you ask for the next one then feel free to apply that hard, unyielding implement to more sensitive areas. That's right, right there at the very bottom of your ass where your thigh begins. Right up against the inner thigh. Right up in between your sensitive soaking labia, right up against your hard, hurting clit. Ever been cunt spanked before, honey? It's happening now, and keep those legs wide for it, keep that ass arched out. Keep the cadence, honey.

"Thank you for making me be a good girl, sir. Please may I have another?" Smack.

Oh yes, honey, every red mark on your ass now makes up for one on the page. Every red mark now atones for every little notch of less-than-perfect performance. Feel it, feel the catharsis building up. You can cry if you want to, cry in response to the pain, to the humiliation of being bent over and spanked like a bad little girl.

Harder! You can give in to it, feel the tears building up inside.

Harder! It's okay to cry, honey, it's okay to not cry, the only requirement here is that every last smack be taken out on your upturned and by now well punished bottom. So now you're going to finish, you're going to stop reading now and finish off the full measure of punishment. Finish it off honey, do it the way you know it needs to be done. I'm counting on you to be a good girl for me. Finish your spanking before you turn the page.

Part Six

And now we're back, honey, and you're done, with your now very red and sore ass high in the air. It is still in the air, isn't it honey? You didn't get out of position just because you were done, before you were told you could, did you? And you did finish every last spank, didn't you, every last one given hard enough, firm and on target? So what I want now is the make-up spanking, the extra strokes for every one that didn't count, for imperfect posture, for moving, for every transgression not yet redeemed. You know how bad you were, honey, so you know how much more you need. So do it honey, lay them on there, fast and furious. Lay them on until you are done, until your sore, smarting ass has completely atoned for your sins. Ask for each one, honey. Convince me that you need it, convince yourself. I'm watching, I'm waiting, do it, do it now.

Part Six

And now I'm satisfied, honey. I'm convinced that you are one hundred percent good girl now, every last red mark taken off the page and put on your ass. Did you cry after all honey, did the tears come, or did you fight them down, keep control the whole time?

I want to know the answers to those questions, but the more important question is, was it enough for you, honey? Yes you're my good girl now, my well spanked, well loved good girl, but how do you feel inside, do you think you need still more spanking to meet your own standard, or do you think you've had enough? Because this isn't about me, this is about you, and so if you haven't had enough chastisement, if you still feel rebellious in your heart, if you still feel guilty, if you still feel unfinished, then there is only one solution here, and that is more spanking.

Yes, honey, more. And this time it's going to be hard and fast and you aren't going to ask for them, oh no, you're just going to get them, *smack, smack, smack,* until you *are* finished, done, completely, cathartically, thoroughly spanked as much as you need to be spanked. The tears are there honey, whether they come spilling out is up to you because you're the one who needs this, you're the one who's been craving this deep, deep down inside for oh, so very long. So keep it up honey, don't short-change yourself, this is where you get a lasting impression, this is where you truly learn how it's going to be. Keep it up until you feel like you've been put completely, utterly, totally in your place. Harder honey, and faster, and turn the page when you're finally done.

Part Six

And one more smack, honey, one more juicy one right in the centre to finish you off properly, harder than all the others. One last sacrifice on your own sexual altar and then you can just let it go, let your implement of self-inflicted penance drop to the floor and just experience what it's like to be bent over, well punished, humiliated, chastised, bright red ass in the air, waiting for permission to get up.

So, what happens next is the question. You have to understand what's going through my mind as I'm administering this to you. It's hard for me to do it, hard to punish you like this and I want nothing more than to hold you and cuddle you and comfort you, and tell you how much you're my good girl now, how proud I am of you for taking it so well. At the same time my cock is rigid, pressing painfully against the bulged out front of my jeans and it's presenting me with an entirely different priority.

Yeah, honey, with your now bright red ass and creamy cunt so perfectly presented the urge is to just get my cock into you and fuck you, oh, so hard and oh, so deep, while you're in this state of ultimate vulnerability, ultimate receptivity. And the only thing that competes with that, honey, is the sight of your tender little anus peeking out between your well spanked buttocks, and the thought of taking you up that hot, tight little hole, spearing my cock deep between your well punished cheeks, finishing off your humiliation with a thorough ass fucking, with the deep, forced injection of sperm into your helpless, hapless rectum.

Yeah, I want that honey, more than anything, but there's one final option, which is to leave you there on display to absorb the details of the lesson you have just received. A little quiet time in the punishment position to reflect at leisure on your new reality. And you can't quite believe it, honey, that I've got you exactly where I want you. You can't believe I've got you exactly where you've wanted to be for years. But I have you here and I'm going to keep you here and you can expect to grow quite used to this situation. Are you up for that, honey? Is there any possibility that you're going to do anything but sigh in satisfaction at the knowledge that somebody, somewhere, is finally going to be giving you exactly the attention you deserve?

No, honey, there isn't. And you know what? Since you've been such a good girl for me, since you've played the game so well I'm going to give you a little treat, which is to reach back between your spread legs. Yeah, you know what's coming next, don't you? Bad girls get spankings and good girls get their stiff little clits stroked until they feel tingly-nice all over. And I know your clit is stiff honey, I know it's hard, peeking out over your swollen, spanked, spread vulva. I know you're slippery back there, I know how much you need the post-spanking release. So yes, honey-good-girl, yes, you can rub your hot little clit in just that special way. You can let me take care of you just like that. Do it honey, rub it up and down, steady strokes, rub it up and down and gasp and sigh and wiggle and think about the show you're putting on for me while you're doing it. Remember how you felt the first time I watched you? Remember the feeling of my eyes on your ass? Feel that now as you do it, feel that sensation as you get wetter, get hotter. Feel your cunt swell up as it gets juicier. Yes, honey, it's going to happen.

It's going to happen very soon now, and you know that your display is going to remove every option but one from my world, and that is to get my cock into you, to finish claiming your body for my own, so think about that, honey, listen for the slither of my belt coming through the loops and feel your heart skip a beat as you wonder if you're going to get it on the ass again, wonder if maybe the spanking isn't over after all. And feel the relief as you hear the buckle hit the floor and the soft pop-pop-pop of my button fly coming undone, and spread your cunt for it, honey, stretch it wide and open and feel me coming up behind you. Sense the warmth of my body, hear me breathing, feel my hands coming on to your poor red ass cheeks, feel the sharp sting as I lift them and spread them, stretching you wider still. And you have a moment here, honey, to wonder if I'm going to take your ass or your cunt. It's a long moment, honey, and you can take it to focus on the heft and hardness of the shaft that's about to slide into your beautifully displayed body. Oh yes, honey, it's going to be so good. I love making you into my good little girl.

And feel the smooth and swollen head nudge up between your soft folds, feel it slide right up into your cunt in one long, steady thrust. Yes, honey, I'm taking your cunt, and not because I'm not highly motivated to claim your tight little anal ring but because I'm saving that for later. You've been a good girl and your cunt deserves its fucking and right now that's exactly what it's going to get. So feel my hands on your ass, honey, feel my fingers digging in and pulling your hips back on to my cock, feel it swelling inside you, harder still.

God, you're so hot, honey, you're so tight, and there is nothing in my world right now but the sight of my cock, glazed shiny with your juices, pumping up into your tight-stretched twat. There is nothing in my world but the feel of your red welted ass in my hands and the scent of your arousal and your cries of mingled pain and pleasure as I fuck you hard and deep and over and over again. It's going to happen, honey. You're going to come on my cock, you're going to jerk and spasm and cry and your muscles are going to go tight and in that instant I'm going to fill you, drive myself all the way into your clenching pussy and empty my balls into you. That's the way it's supposed to work. You're the woman and I'm the man and your job is to get your ass up and take what I have to give you, and my job is to make sure you get it, get everything you need, in full and overflowing measure. You needed the spanking and you need the fucking and in a little while you're going to need that quiet moment and the time to touch and to look and to wonder at the amazing power of this whole thing, but right now what you need to do is come.

Part Six

That's right, honey. That's right, good girl. Come for me, come on me, keep that steady rhythm on your clit and feel my cock inside you. Feel so claimed, so taken, so open and exposed and receptive, all dignity, all defences, everything but your most fundamental feminine nature stripped and discarded to reveal the most primal, beautiful, natural you. And there is nothing in this world you want more than to feel me come inside you, hear me grunt and groan and feel my cock swell and stiffen, even longer and thicker than it is right now, stretching you to the point of pain and throbbing, pulsing, drenching your open, fertile womb with my sperm. There's nothing you want more than that, and in order to get it you have to come yourself, so come on honey, show me what a good girl you are, show me that you know what to do. Come for me. Do it. Do it right now. Now now *now NOW*!

And, oh yes, honey, you get your reward for that. You get my cock thrust up inside you so deep it feels like you're going to be torn in half and you get my hands clenched on your sore, spanked ass and your legs forced even wider. You get slammed hard and deep and you get my everything, not just my balls but my very being, my passion, my desire, my very soul pumped up inside you, completing you, completing me.

You get it all honey, and you get me pulling you down, off whatever it is you're bent over to lie with me in a tangled heap on the floor, the couch, the bed, whatever, wherever. You get me inside you still hard, drenched in sweat and you get to forget about everything but the intimacy of this contact and the feel of me behind you and inside you. You get me reaching around to hold you, to cup your breasts with surprising gentleness, to kiss the back of your neck, to whisper to you.

You're such a good girl.

You get that, good girl. You get everything, because you are you and I am me and that's the way it's meant to be.

Bike Girl

Leather, heavy and black, zipped on like a second skin. It makes me wet just to smell it. Boots on, gloves on, my hair tied back and then helmet on. I mount up, start up, feel the vibration in my crotch, steady, insistent. Hit the gas, pop the clutch and I'm riding, Harley hot, rolling past the stop signs on my quiet suburban street, past my disapproving neighbours, past the oversized houses on undersized lots, the mass-market McMansions that crowd my executive ghetto. Every one is a unique design, exclusive, builder customized to buyer specifications. Every one is exactly the same with its manicured lawn and cathedral entrance and designer-styled kitchen.

I cruise past the grandiose clubhouse of the golf course that narrowly squiggles its way through everyone's back yard so everyone can claim to have a golf course lot. It spills pretentious music into the street, and I cut too close to a grey haired foursome crossing the street to whatever dinner party is being held there tonight. They jump, and I smirk behind my facemask at their blurred annoyance. Fuck them, smug, safe, pretentious post-love-child yuppie sellouts. I don't stop at the stop sign, just slow enough to clear left and right and then punch it, out onto the main drag, from nearly zero to way-too-fast in too few seconds to count. My heart rate spikes with the tach, the engine screams and the wind roars as the speedometer races from warning to fine to vehicular homicide. I take her down the yellow line, away from the subdivision, away from prestige and position and status and into the gathering darkness.

They'd ban me if they could, that smug foursome and my neighbours and the rest of my snobby little world. They'd pen a covenant to deny the ownership of motorcycles in our tight-assed little might-as-well-be-gated community. Only they never thought of tuned headers and dual carbs and the sweet rumble-roar of two hundred hard-ridden Harley horses, and whoever drew up the original rules wasn't as smart as I am. They aren't going to make any changes that I choose to oppose, the clauses don't allow it. I fight dirty and I always win, and I can feel myself become a creature of the night as the big, round moon breaks over the horizon. It's a werewolf-worthy transformation, power-suited power lawyer to black leather biker bitch, and my blood is boiling with the change. My fertility peaks when the moon is full, and fuck I'm so horny I could rip a man's throat out for access to his cock.

I jump into the other lane to blow past a sensibly driven Volvo and feel the rush of speed. I'm naked under the tight, restraining leather, with the engine throbbing against my clit while my nipples rub on my jacket, rigid hard. I'm a machine-melded sex-goddess, as steamy as the Amazon and twice as hot. Already my womb is pulsing in anticipation of power-driven climax, the real reason for my ride.

Oh yes, I want it, I want it so bad I can barely see straight and I'm sure my driving judgment is impaired by my arousal and so what if it is? And you might think I'd be at home waiting for my husband to come and scratch the full-moon itch, but I never let him touch me when I'm ripe like this. Ovulation week belongs to my bike. I tell him it's the rhythm method, but it's really automotive adultery.

I slide around the parkway curve and will the traffic lights to be green. Amber flashes instead and I gun it, clear left, clear right and blast through the lights at twice the legal limit. And yes, that could get me killed and you should ask me if I care. The full moon makes me crazy, or maybe I was just born that way. For a split second I think I see blue-red-blue roof lights and adrenaline spikes for the chase, but it's just some pizza driver with a lighted logo on his car. *Party Pizza for your Pizza Party.*

The thought crosses my mind that I could nail the brakes, wave him over, flip up the faceplate and suck him off in the ditch. He'd get a story no-one would ever believe, and I'd get two minutes with some loser's cock in my mouth and then a face-full of Party Pizza special sauce. I'd get dirtied, and then I'd ride with the faceplate up, to let his juice dry on my pretty-girl features, to let it mix with road grime so when I came back to my husband I was streaked with the evidence of my infidelity. The thought makes my clit throb hard. Oh yes, I want to be dirtied, I want it bad. And by the time the thought is finished pizza-guy is a mile in my dust and I'm spinning up the on-ramp. I shift up as I hit the highway, slide to the fast lane and wind her out.

Wind her *right* out as the dashed lines flicker past in a hypnotic blur, way over the speed limit. My thoughts turn to a square shouldered cop with handcuffs and a nightstick and a willingness to trade violation for violation. I picture myself cuffed, bent over the hood of his cruiser, engine heat burning my cheek, black leather down around my knees as he slam fucks my ass, first with the nightstick, then with a cock that makes the stick look small by comparison.

Involuntarily my thighs clench on the saddle and I get close to the edge, so very close. My concentration is split exactly in two, half on the road, half on my clenching cunt. I have to slow down as I get hotter or risk a fatal wipeout, but it's the speed that turns me on. The result is an excruciatingly drawn out approach to orgasm, an advanced form of machine masturbation that guarantees a mind-wiping climax, torqued even tighter by the fact that even as I lose control of my body I have to keep control of the bike. One day I'm not going to do that. One day I'm going to hit the gas when the pleasure-wave hits me, and then just let it take me away, give myself to my bike completely, and to the concrete five seconds later. I don't care if death hurts, so long as it's fast.

And fast is what it's about. I ramp up the speed and visualize the cop-cock impaling me, lifting my feet off the ground with every stroke into my overstretched ass as he punishes me for my transgression of velocity. I long to reach down and touch my clit, but at this speed I can't take my hands off the handlebars. In my mind he's getting harder, longer, thicker as his own explosion approaches, his hands digging painfully into my hips as he violates me over and over. I am completely trapped between his powerful thighs and the hood of the cruiser and he smacks my ass and makes me say, "Please fuck me, I'm a bad girl."

"Please fuck me, I'm a bad girl." I can feel his cock twitch when I say it and I say it again reflexively, because he likes it, because I want him to come inside me, to empty his huge balls into my aching rectum, because I am a bad girl, a very bad girl, and I do so need to be dirtied like this, knocked off my Manolo Blahniks, torn out of my Chanel suit, and put very thoroughly in my place. I long to be reduced to my cunt and made to grovel for sex, and if that sounds politically incorrect to you, well, you need a different book.

"Please fuck me, I'm a bad girl." I say it out loud to myself, as the bike finds my rhythm. "Please fuck me, I'm a bad girl." I can feel my anus clenching around his imaginary cock, feel the heat of humiliation on my cheeks, and most of all feel my Harley's steady throb against my pulsing clit. I slow down to keep control, to lose control, and focus my mind on the feel of cold metal cuffs on my wrists. "Please fuck me, I'm a bad girl. Please make it hard, please make it hurt, please fill me up with cock, with cum, with degradation." The rumble of the engine finds my sweetspot. "Please make me feel it, make me take it, make me dirty, make me yours."

And I'm trembling now with the intensity and I have to shift to the slow lane. In my mind the cop's hands find my tits, clamping down on my nipples to give me what I'm begging for. Pain explodes through them and my cunt gushes in response. I don't know why my fantasy life is so dark, so violent, and I don't care. The leather of my riding pants is riding up in my crotch, putting pressure right where I need it as I rock my hips against the seat. He has me now, his cock is an iron bar sliding in so hard and deep and I am bent over in ritual supplication, my ass split and presented and penetrated. I am helpless, so open, so taken, so completely, utterly possessed by this man and all I want is more. I want him to destroy me with his cock and that's exactly what he's doing, inch by inch by inch.

Fuck yes. I have to fight to keep my eyes from rolling back in my head, have to slow down again, and the engine's screaming roar is now a steady purr, just enough to tease me in steady rhythm. *Fuck yes.* My clit is pulsing, and every muscle in my body is rigid as I squirm against the vibrations. And I imagine him coming, pumping his sperm deep into my sore, punished ass with hard, aggressive thrusts, swelling thick enough to spike pain through my already overstretched sphincter. The head is so big it won't actually come out. He and I are tied together like mating dogs, locked in sex until he is finished with me, though his overflowing juice is already dribbling down my ass cheeks.

That last image does it and I come, hard, convulsing on the seat, screaming in my helmet, my hands locked rigid on the handlebars and thank god this section of road is straight. I can feel my cunt clenching, gushing, anointing the crotch of my riding pants with slippery sex. The orgasm goes on forever and it seems like I'll never stop. Finally it dies away in a succession of ever smaller contractions, the waves of pleasure leaving my body limp and trembling. My faceplate is fogged up and I flip it up to feel the wind on my face. The inside of my leathers are soaked in sweat, and on my face it cools and dries, reminding me of my first, fast, pizza-boy fantasy.

I unzip my jacket enough to let the night air in and the sudden chill stiffens my already erect nipples to painful sensitivity. They rub against the rough leather, sending aftershocks through my overstimulated system. There's no sex like the solo ride. My husband is a good man in every sense, a hard worker, a provider, on his way up in his firm. I enjoy our intimacy and he treats me like a princess, but he can't make me feel the way my Harley does.

I take a few deep breaths to recover and as I do, I pass a dark shape on the center median. It's a cop, lurking there in the night with his radar. I'm going too slowly now to catch his interest, and I laugh that my fantasy has spared me from the reality of a speeding stop. The pizza-boy vision replays in my mind, this time with the radar cop in his place. This cop isn't the poster boy stud I was conjuring up a minute ago but a three hundred pound donut pig, with his belly overlapping his gunbelt. In sixty fast seconds of mind-fucking myself I make him have a heart attack even as he comes on my face, and I leave him dead by the roadside with his pants around his ankles. Call me sick if you want, I just might like it.

Gear up and back to cruising speed. I've noticed something about my ovulation week dreams. The sex is always degrading, but when the degradation is because the man is a loser its oral sex and I'm the one calling the shots. When the guy is a stud then he takes my cunt or my ass and I have no control at all. The first kind gets me hot, but it's the second kind that gets me off. You might try to dig some deep psychological meaning out of that. Good luck to you.

I accelerate a little more as a sign flashes overhead. I've chosen my route unconsciously, heading in to the sky glow of the city. The post orgasmic bliss doesn't last long, and I need to find more excitement. A minute later excitement finds me. Someone blows past on a red/black blur that might have been a

Kawasaki Ninja. Instinctively I hit the gas to race him, then I remember the speed trap. No way this guy didn't light up the radar gun. I glance over my shoulder and see blue-red-blue flashing, coming fast. I maintain speed, wait for the cop to come flying past and then fall in behind him, winding out the revs to keep up. Ninja-boy is running, and this cop intends to make quota tonight.

And me? I'm getting a free ride with the speedo up in the stupid part of the dial. My path is being cleared by blue-red-blue, and any cop ahead of me is going to be deployed to stop the Ninja. It's my own private police escort and the wind is almost lifting me right out of my seat. My adrenaline surges as the chase eats up mileage. There's no traffic, no nothing, it's fucking beautiful. Too soon brake lights flare and the cop pulls over to the left. The Ninja has gotten away. I slow down to sanity, pass the cop as he turns around at the crossover, going back the way he came, then throttle up again.

The adrenaline and the speed have got me juiced up once more, and I think about the Ninja rider chasing me down and slicing the crotch of my leathers open with a hunting knife so he can fuck me over the seat of my still running bike. He's tall and dark and strong and he knows exactly what he's doing. Yeah, my rape imagery always involves guys who I'd fuck in a heartbeat, so is that really rape? My clit throbs as I run the fantasy, but traffic picks up as I come into downtown and I can't focus enough to make it happen. Instead I weave the traffic, grab an offramp into the wrong side of town. Spray painted buildings, boarded up windows, trash on the street corners, some of it wearing gang colors.

Angry eyes follow me and I don't stop for the red lights that still work. The fantasy morphs into a gang bang, anonymous young faces with hard eyes, my clothing torn off, my arm twisted painfully behind me, my face shoved down on dirty pavement while I'm fucked by a succession of anonymous inner-city cocks, each eager to take class vengeance on upper-crust suburban cunt. I squirm in my seat, feel the engine throb, but I'm not going anywhere near fast enough with city driving, and this place carries the very real risk of turning my fantasy into reality. All I'd have to do to make that happen is stop, but I'm not quite that self destructive, not tonight anyway. I need to get back on the highway.

And then a red-black Ninja cruises past and I lock eyes with the rider, and realize it's not Ninja Boy but Ninja Girl, blonde and hot in her leather and on a whim, on a compulsion, I pull a one-eighty and follow. I'm a Harley rider and I won't give the time of day to someone who pilots Kawasaki scrap, but I only know one woman who would race the cops like that, and that's me. Maybe it's my competitive instinct, maybe it was the way her eyes burned in to mine as we passed, but I follow her, not too close, not too far back. She leads me out of the bad area into downtown proper, still a place you could get mugged or murdered, but here it isn't a given. She parks in front of a trendy nightclub and walks up a side street. I park and follow her.

The place she turns into is a blank storefront. Above the door is a number, twenty-three-seventeen. The windows are frosted white glass, and one of them bears the etched black outline of an old fashioned key. There's no other marking, no indication of what might lie behind the door. I hesitate, then try the handle. It opens. Inside is a vestibule, a set of stairs leading down, the faint pulse of music. It's a club of some kind. The woman from the Ninja has taken off her leather jacket, is handing it to a coat check girl whose look is too hardcore to be simply affected goth. She takes something in exchange, a snaky riding crop. She looks up, our eyes meet, my knees go weak. Fantasy is becoming reality. My life is about to change

Part Seven

Yeah you know the Club, don't you, honey? That's the Club where Julie went to start her advanced classes. That's the Club where the trainer polished his skills, where cage-girl is displayed, where the traveller comes when he comes home. You know what bike-girl is going to find there, don't you? You know what's behind that door she's just stepped through, because it's your door, my door, our door, and every time you see a door you're reminded of me, reminded of the desire I ignite in you. Every time you see a door you can't help knowing that I'm just on the other side of it, just that close to you.

Bike-girl's highway is our road, her journey is our connection and in a very real way, she is you. Believe it, honey. You're both united in your need for that burning consummation, so lacking in your normal life. You know it because you can feel it out there, waiting for you, and you desire it, you need it, you want it. That's why you come to me, isn't it, honey? You want it hard, you want it dirty. I know you don't want to ask for it that way. That would be so much harder, wouldn't it, honey? It would be so embarrassing, so humiliating to come right out and say what it is you've been craving for so very long. So I'm going to make it easy on you, honey, and I'm just going to give it to you. You don't have to ask for it, beg for it, plead for it. You can even protest if you want, you can struggle, you can fight. You can do anything you want, just so long as when you're done you do what I want you to do. And you know you're going to honey, just like I know you're going to, because deep down we both know what you need.

So what I want you to do, honey, is go and get your favourite midnight friend, you know the one I mean, that firm, phallic shaft that does it for you when no-one else is going to, the one that violated your open holes while you did your homework like Julie. You're going to get fucked soon honey, you're going to get fucked hard and deep and there's nothing you can do about it, nothing you can say. This won't be a fantasy, this is going to be as real as it gets, and we both know how your belly tightens up when I say that.

And I just want to say, while you remember where it is you put your favourite masturbation tool, that I love doing this to you, I love reaching out and touching you like this, I love the fact that you'll do everything I want you to do, even when you can't admit you want it. Even when you really don't want

Part Seven

it. Ooops, did I say that, honey? How very politically incorrect of me. A post-millenium man who prefers smart, accomplished, independent women shouldn't ever think of making them do things they don't want to do, should he? He most certainly shouldn't like it.

But I do like it, honey, and so do you, and that's not a contradiction because there are different ways of *wanting it* and even though you might not like what's happening, you like the fact that it's happening anyway. You want that, you need that, because it means you're not in control. And you do need to be out of control, don't you, honey? Say "Yes," for me. You know enough to say that by now.

"Yes, I want to be out of control."

"Yes, I'm going to do whatever you want me to."

And so you can start by stopping, honey, stop right here and go get your cock substitute, because I don't want to wait any longer. Just do it, do it now.

Part Seven

Oh yes, honey, feel it in your hand, long and thick and firm. You know where it's going, don't you? Or at least you think you do. I'll tell you right now you've got part of the answer. Does your heart race when you read that, honey? Do you get a little hotter, breathe a little faster when you think about what the other part might be?

Yes, you do, I know you do. So what I want you to do is kiss it honey, kiss the very tip of that rigid shaft. Run your tongue around it; lick it like ice-cream. Lick it like it was my cock. You want more now, you want to feel it sliding into your mouth, parting your lips, opening you, putting you into that sexually receptive position, that sexually receptive state. I want you to know something, honey, and that is that my cock is rigid for you right now. It's as hard as that shaft in your hand, as the one that your soft, supple lips are making love to right now. I want you to picture that now, picture my cock with just a drop of fluid glistening at its tip. Realize how warm it is, how hard and how soft at the same time. Take in the swollen, purple head and realize how it's going to make you feel to be down on your knees in front of it, looking up at me looking down as you go to work to earn a face full of sperm. Yeah, work it honey, work it hard for me.

And slide that shaft right in to your mouth, one firm, deep motion, slide it as far as it can go and then hold it there. Use your lips, use your tongue, that's the deal, that's the ideal. You want it to feel so good for me, right honey? And now that you're sucking on it, we'll just relax and have a little chat.

How was your day, honey? How was your week? Was it long? Was it stressful? Did you have to deal with too much from too many people? I know you managed it, I know you came out on top. You're so good at what you do, honey, I'm proud of you.

Keep sucking honey, I didn't say to stop.

Now think about the last good book you read, think about the title. I'd love to talk to you about it, have a nice, long, intimate conversation about it. I'd love to hear what you have to say.

Except of course you don't have anything to say right now, because your mouth is full of cock. So let's not think, let's just experience. And what I want you to experience is that violating phallus stroking in and out, all the way in, and all the way out, over and over and over again. Do that for me, fuck your mouth the way I'd fuck it. Do it hard and long and keep on doing it. I want your lips to be sore, I want your jaw to ache, I want your entire world to become my cock, and that's the only thing that's going to happen. I want it to be uncomfortable. I want it to be awkward and humiliating. I want you to feel like a degraded little slut, face-fucking herself on command, on my command.

Are you going to do that for me? Are you going to be my eager, willing little slut? Keep that cock moving honey, that's the only answer I need. Keep it going in and out. It's making you wet, isn't it honey? It's making your eager little pussy juice to be forced into this, and the more uncomfortable it is the more you want it.

Oh yes, you want it underlined that you're not the one in charge here, that your job here is just to take whatever it is I have to give to you. Go on, suck it harder, honey, suck it like you mean it. You want to show me how good you are, don't you? You want to show me how much better you are at this than all the other girls. You want to be the dirtiest, the nastiest, the sluttiest. You want to turn me on so much, get me so hard that I have no choice but to grab your head and slam fuck your mouth until I jet my sperm into you and onto you. And then you're going to look up at me with this expression halfway between innocence and decadence with your face all flushed and dripping with sperm. And you know just how hot you'll look in that moment, and you know the best way to get that look is just to get into it, to be that dirty, that slutty, that depraved. And so you're doing it, and you don't need me to tell you to suck harder, but you like it when I do because then you know you're doing it for me.

Suck harder. Yeah, you get to me. I have no trouble telling you that. Fuck yes, suck it you hot little slut, suck it cunt, come on, show me you deserve to have your face sprayed. Fuck yes, do it for me, get into it, feel the head of my cock at the back of your throat as confirmation of just how good you are. Fuck yes, feel my balls tighten up, inhale the scent of me, rich and masculine, taste me, taste the proof of my desire as it leaks out on your tongue. You can feel it coming, feel me coming and you want it, more than anything, that salty, sticky stamp of approval, and the feeling of satisfaction, of completion, that comes with it. Oh, fuck yes, you want it and I want it, honey, and I am thrusting my hips, forcing it between your lips as you suck and you are exactly where you want to be with your lips wrapped around my cock and you know what's going to happen next.

Or maybe you don't. Because what I want to see now is that shaft coming out of your mouth and going up your tight, wet cunt right now. Now! Now*now*now! Just fucking do it, get it in, I don't care if you're ready for it or not. Don't ease it in, don't tease it, just slide it right up there because I want you to feel violated, honey. I want you to feel taken and right out of control. Right up there, until you're stuffed full, stretched as wide as you can go, and then start fucking yourself with it. Just do it, and I know I don't have to worry that you aren't wet enough because you're fucking soaked.

Say, "Yes," honey. Your mouth isn't full of cock now.
Say it again. "Yes."
Say it again. "Yes." Say it every stroke.
"Yes. Yes. Yes. Yes."
"YesyesyesYES!"
"Yes, oh yes, oh my fucking god, yes, please *YES!*"

Part Seven

Do it fucking harder, do it slutty, make it raw, make it hurt. In and out and in and out and thrust your hips up to get it deeper. Take it to the hilt, to your womb, and feel your clit swell up in response. Grunt and groan and wiggle on it, wriggle on it. Degrade yourself with it, display yourself, release yourself, reduce yourself to a screaming ball of flesh and sex. This isn't about foreplay, this isn't about romance, this is about deep depravity. Show me you're the hottest bitch in the world. Put yourself on show, get my attention, take my attention, make it impossible for me to look anywhere other than at you, at your body, at what you're doing to yourself, and to me. Make it so that wherever I go, whatever I do, I'll be unable to forget this moment, unable to get the image of this wanton sex vixen spreading herself, fucking herself, debasing herself for me. Give me a show so hot no other woman can hope to compete, give me everything, utterly. Oh yes, honey. Fuck your hot little pussy for me, clench it down, squeeze it tight, gasp and moan and show me how good it's going to feel when I get into your cunt. Show me you can do it better than anyone. Show me that for me you have no limits.

Fucking do it, and know that you're burning yourself into my brain with this, know that I will never forget this moment as long as I live. Feel my eyes on you, on your body, on your open, spread cunt. Can you feel my arousal, boiling now in the flame of your sex? Remember how hard my cock was a second ago, forcing your lips apart? It's harder now, honey. Oh yeah, spread your cunt for me, lick your fingers and rub your clit. Get your fingers slippery and then lick them clean, slow and sexy. Yeah that's right. Make it good for me. Now get your fingers slippery again and smear your face with your juices. Show me what a dirty girl you are. Slick them up again and smear your tits. Do it again. Coat yourself in sex. Fuck, you're such a hot slut. My hot slut. You are so mine, you're mine everywhere, aren't you, slut? Aren't you, bitch?

Yes, you *are* mine, everywhere. You know what's coming next, honey. Slide that slippery shaft out of your wide stretched pussy and slide it down, down between your round, ripe ass cheeks. Feel the thrill as the tip slides over your tight little rosebud. Oh yes, honey. You're mine everywhere. So push it now, gently, firmly, steadily, rhythmically. Oh yeah, open up your secret hole for me. Push it in, so deep and hard, opening you right up. I'm going to watch you violate your ass. Get it it, and once it's in, get it moving in and out. Fuck, that's hot, I can see your cunt contract every time you push in. Do it, do it, *do it*. In, out, *in, out, in, in, IN!*

And yes, honey, I know it's uncomfortable, and yes, honey, I know it's degrading and yes, honey, that's exactly why I'm making you do it, because I want you uncomfortable and I want you degraded because I want all of you, even this part. I want to know there's nothing you won't do for me. I want to know that I can have you anytime, anywhere, any way I want, and every way I want. Get it in honey, get it in deeper, you know I want it. Get it in honey, get it in hard.

Oh fuck, yes. I just love the expression on your face when it goes in deeper, mingled pain and pleasure and most of all surrender, sweet surrender. Every woman has defences, she has to, but yours are gone now, washed away as you display for me, as you sodomize yourself for me, as you do your level best to show me that no other woman can possibly be what you're willing to be for me. Deeper honey, I want to see it all the way in, driven right up your tight little rectum. I want to see you struggle to take it all. Yeah, you're my everything now, my sweet-sucking slut, my easy, sleazy, eager beaver, my hot little anal whore. Fucking do it. And I don't have to ask if this is turning you on, I can see it in the rigid pulse of your clit, in the cunt-contractions that happen every time that shaft goes in. You need to be assfucked now, so say it.

"Yes sir, I need to be assfucked."

Say it again, honey.

"Yes sir, I need to be assfucked."

And oh yes, that's good to hear, that gets my cock so hard. But I'm not sure I believe you, honey, so it until you've convinced me it's true.

Yes sir, please fuck my tight little ass."

Say it until you've convinced yourself.

"Yes sir, please sir I need it so bad. Yes sir, please sir, please let me please you. Please let me show you how good it will be, and please sir, please, please fuck my tight little ass."

And yeah, you want it, you need to feel it, feel my cock violating you over and over again. You want, you need, you crave the feeling, the hot wet gush of my sperm deep, deep inside. You need to feel me to claim your very soul as my stiff shaft swells, as it stiffens until you think you're going to be torn in half. Yeah, you want that, and you would come in a heartbeat if I let you. You know you have to have permission, right, honey? You know those are the rules. So come on, honey, convince me you need to come.

"Yes sir, I need to come."

Fuck it.

"Please sir, let me come with your cock up my ass."

Fuck it hard.

"Please sir, I'm so hot for you."

Take it deep.

"Please sir, I'm your little anal slut. I'm being so good for you. Please sir, look at me assfuck myself just to turn you on. Please sir, I need it so bad, I'm such a dirty girl for you."

Fucking do it, hard and fast.

"Please sir, I'm yours, completely yours. Take me, fuck me, hurt me, do anything you want to me, but please, please, please let me come for you."

Part Seven

Oh yeah, honey, I love watching you like this, watching your eyes get desperate for it. Rub your clit honey. Rub it hard, and keep on fucking your ass. Fuck, I love the way you can't help but hump it. Fuck, I love the way you grovel and beg with your body. Fuck, I love having you like this.

And you love it too, don't you honey? You love being my degraded little slut, you love going where no other woman would go.

"Yes sir, I love it. Yes sir, thank you, sir, for making me be your dirty little anal slut."

And yes honey, now you can come. Now you can finally get your fingers going on your hot little clit, on your spread and juicy cunt, you can rub it hard and fast while the overwhelming urge to release builds up in your body. See how tight your nipples have gotten, aching, pointing, swollen on their own. More to the point, see how deeply your mind is engaged, see how completely I've swept you up in this rawest of raw sex acts, see how completely I've carried you away. You're mine, completely mine and that building orgasm is your physical signature on that basic fact. So do it, honey. Climaxfor me, give me your body the way I've taken your mind. Do it hard, make it slutty, make it intense, make it impossible for me to look away and just fucking do it. Do it fucking hard and fucking deep, scream it, pump it, make it, take it,

Oh yes. Fuck, you make me so hard.

Bike Girl II

Ninja Girl holds my gaze, and I am captivated like a cobra facing a mongoose, all my lethal self-assuredness drained by the sight of my nemesis. Another woman is standing behind a counter, black hair, black corset, pale skin, with an ankh hanging from a black leather necklace between her breasts. Her face looks fragile, but her body is lithe and muscular.

"Who are you with?" The pale girl is the doorkeeper, her question is casual, standard, but she's serious about it.

"I'm…" I want to lie, to get in to this suddenly fascinating place. Except I have no lie to tell, I'm not with anyone, and I'm not going to be admitted, and the fantasy that had started to weave itself around Ninja Girl and her riding crop dissolves.

"She's with me." Ninja Girl's eyes hold mine as she comes to my rescue. She wants to ensnare me in something deeper and I feel my face flush at the prospect.

"Okay." The doorkeeper sits down and my saviour, my captor beckons me over.

"Give her your jacket." She motions to the girl behind the coat check, this one in a black miniskirt, black fishnets with red high heels and a black bra, nothing else. I feel a rush of arousal flood through my system. I've heard about places like this. I've never been to one.

"But I'm not wearing anything..."

"Give her your jacket." Her tone is calm, commanding. Wordlessly I unzip my jacket, expose my naked breasts. I hesitate a moment, my heart pounding, while her eyes burn into mine. I surrender, look down, shrug the jacket off and hand it across the counter, standing there half naked. The girl gives me a claim check that I have nowhere to put. Ninja Girl takes it, the symbolism lost on neither of us, and suddenly my pulse is pounding in my temples. My nipples have risen in the sudden coolness, and my excitement with them. All at once I want nothing more than for this anonymous stranger to kiss me, but she doesn't. I feel a stab of rejection, and the desire shifts, to have her grab my vulnerable, exposed nipples and twist, to have her slap me across the face, to have her grab my hair and force me to the dirty floor. That little mind-flip probably means something deep about me, and in it a good therapist might find the deeper reasons behind my moonlight rides and the violent sex that they boil up from my soul.

Except there's no therapist here, though Ninja Girl might yet excise my possessing demons. My eyes slide down from hers, it doesn't seem to be my place to meet her gaze. Instead I focus on the tip of her riding crop, black and menacing, a symbol of power. I find myself wishing she'd just use it on me now and spare me the suspense, but she doesn't do any of the things my twisted little mind desires her to do. Instead she turns and goes down the stairs. I hesitate but follow her. The stairs are long, and the music grows louder as we descend. At the bottom is a door, and a short corridor, and another door, and behind it…

Behind it is decadence. The room is dark, dim lit with neon squiggles of red and blue. Three couples fuck on a wrestling mat, bodies intertwined, undulating like sex crazed snakes, glistening slick with sprayed-on oil. Beyond them a naked woman is locked in a set of stocks, her mouth gagged open, a mechanized, flywheel driven phallus driving into her from behind, deep, powerful, rhythmic. It glistens with her juices, obscenely distending her cunt with every penetration, and her eyes are rolled back in her head, caught between anguish and nirvana. There's a dance floor full of grinding bodies in various stages between leather and naked, and some of them are fucking, too. A redhead with a whip sits spread-legged in a throne-like chair while a blonde kneels submissively between her thighs, lapping at her cunt with adoration in her eyes. My head swims and I feel faint, the rush of my pulse now loud enough to compete with the driving beat.

"Here." Ninja Girl points to a padded bench. Three women kneel there already. They're blindfolded, their lips are parted, their fingers are interlaced at the back of their necks. They look like they've been waiting awhile, and their expressions are strangely serene in this anything-but-relaxing environment.

I kneel beside them and lace my fingers in the back of my own neck. The motion raises and presents my breasts, and I wait for the blindfold. Ninja Girl gestures with the riding crop, and hands appear from behind me to take away my vision. The world disappears into darkness, and my other senses heighten to compensate. The pounding beat fills my head, but I can suddenly feel the body heat of the women next to me, I catch the raw scent of female arousal. I sense the movement of people in front of me, behind me. A hand touches my breast and I start, but I don't move from my imposed position. The hand explores, weighing my flesh, testing my firmness, squeezing my nipples to test their responsiveness. I'm proud of my breasts, firm and high set as they are, and this intimate examination is somehow both degrading and exalting.

And it's certainly arousing. My breathing gets short and my clit stiffens as I wet the already soaked crotch of my leathers one more time. My mind drifts away, surrendering to the anonymous hands, though I know somehow it is Ninja Girl who is touching me.

The hands go away and I wait for a timeless time, so long that I begin to worry that my husband will wonder where I've gone. I should call him. I should stop just to let him know that I'm still alive, but I find myself unable to unlace my hands, unable to get up. I remember the peaceful look on the other women's faces and I realize that my own expression must now be similar, my lips parted, an expression of calm resignation on my pretty features. I feel that way, and yet beneath that my heart races like my bike at top revs. My cunt drips steadily, split by my leathers in this position, my nipples stiffen until they hurt, but I don't move, I barely even breathe. My arousal is like the invisible bubbles built up in a bottle of chilled champagne, giving no clue to the pressure contained until it explodes in frothy ecstasy at its uncorking. I want to be uncorked, I want to explode for Ninja Girl, yield myself up to her, give her everything until I am consumed, drained, and if she then casts me aside like an empty bottle, I will accept that as my natural fate. I want the realization of all my throbbing Harley fantasies, I want to be sacrificed at last to the swollen full moon. I want everything, and yet I'm not even sure what *everything* will mean here. I realize in that vision I don't even know her name. Time passes and my arms grow sore from their position, and then my knees, and then my back, and yet still I don't want it to end.

Eventually the music stops. Voices rise, then fade, silence. I wait, aware of the breathing of the women next to me. Someone moves, and then I feel hands, once more on my breasts, tweaking the nipples hard enough to hurt, hard enough to make me gasp, and then they move to my leather riding pants, undo the belt, undo the zipper, slide them down over my hips.

The hands probe at my cunt, parting my labia with sure, strong movements, peeling back the hood from my rigid clit. I can feel rubber gloves on them, and that only fires my imagination, and the clinical distance they add to the process increases my humiliation. The hands cup my buttocks and squeeze, hard, then part them expose my anus. A finger slick with my own juices finds it, slides in, violating me with casual ease. The tight muscle contracts reflexively, and my clit jumps as my heart rate spikes. Some distant part of my mind wonders at how easily I have been objectified, intimately, impersonally inspected by a total stranger I haven't even seen. And yet that same part of my mind understands exactly why this is happening, how this reality fits exactly with my dark, violent fantasy life. I have been needing this for a long time, and now, by accident or fate, I have it.

Reflexively I moan and push back against the invading finger, opening myself to its systematic degradation. Too soon it's withdrawn. I hear the rustle and snap as whoever is wearing the rubber gloves removes them, and perhaps puts on another pair. More sounds come from beside me, a feminine whimper, a gasp, a moan.

We are being tested, my nameless sisters and I. My suspicion is confirmed when a male voice says. "This one."

"Of course," answers Ninja Girl. The male voice was deep, resonant, calm, casual, as if accustomed to being presented with a line of eager sluts. Ninja Girl's response supports the idea that this is true. But which one is *this one*? I dare to hope that it might be me, though I have no idea what being chosen will mean. Excitement still shoots through me, engorging my cunt anew, tightening my nipples to still harder erection, stiffening my clit. And then someone puts their head close to mine, lips grazing my ear, breath hot against my neck. "Do you want more?" The voice is barely a whisper, but I recognize Ninja Girl, and it's like she was reading my mind.

I try to answer but my words catch in my throat. I manage to nod my head. *Yes.*

Her hands find my chin, pull my jaw open, and something goes into my mouth, forcing it open. Straps buckle around the back of my head, holding it in place. I taste rubber, explore with my tongue, find a rubber coated ring holding my jaw wide. It's big enough around to accept quite a sizeable cock, if someone chooses to use me that way. It's big enough around that my jaw aches under the strain already. The hands move on, and a stiff, heavy collar is buckled around my neck. My wrists are cuffed behind me, and my riding pants stripped the rest of the way off. A rope is run from the wrist cuffs to the floor, attached there somehow, and tightened, pulling my shoulders back and pushing my breasts out and up. I have become a sexual package, ready to be express delivered to my new owner.

"She needs to be broken." The voice is the man's, and a thrill of sudden rebellion shoots through me. *No, I don't need to be broken!*

"Of course," Ninja Girl replies.

I try to protest but the ring gag renders intelligible speech impossible. Trussed as I am I can't even struggle, and suddenly I'm afraid. Despite my harsh fantasies, my experience of sex has always been loving and gentle. *I don't need to be broken. I don't want it.*

But it's going to happen. Something, another rope, pulls the ring-gag's harness up, pulling my head up, straightening my posture. My position is taut, caught between the rope on my wrists pulling down and the one on the harness pulling up. I have no idea what's happened to the other women who had been beside me, but I sense that they're gone. *I don't need to be broken!* Another rope goes around each knee, pulling them wide, increasing the tension in my body even further. I'm kneeling, open, helpless, completely vulnerable, and it's far too late for me to exert any influence on the course of events. What's going to happen is going to happen. I try to cry out and I can't, panic rising in my heart. Sex games are one thing, this is something else. Effective protest is impossible, but I jerk and wriggle and make an inarticulate approximation to "No!" What happens is going to happen, but I don't have to go along with it gracefully.

What happens is a line of pain burned across my left breast, right across the nipple. Belatedly I register the *whoosh* and *snap* of what must have been Ninja Girl's riding crop. I howl, something the ring gag doesn't prevent, and another stroke burns itself into my right breast. The pain is unbelievable and my instinct is to fight, to run, to curl up in a ball, anything to protect my most tender flesh from the punishment applied. I can do nothing, and more strokes scourge my tits, steady and systematic, covering them completely. They move to my belly, to the front of my thighs, then, most cruelly, to cut up between my legs to chastise my cunt.

The tip of the riding crop finds my clit and I am nearly blinded by the pain, tears now welling from my eyes. It strikes me there again and I'm sobbing openly. *I don't need to be broken!* Whether I need it or not, it's happening. I scream and try to beg through the cruel gag as the crop comes down, fighting against the restraints to no avail. The steady punishment continues, striping my inner thighs, burning the cheeks of my ass, cutting up between them to punish my pussy, and the tight ring of my anus. The burning streaks fade and blur into one all-encompassing ache, refreshed each time the crop comes down, and finally I am too exhausted to scream to struggle, even to cry, and I just hang there, accepting my fate because I have no choice.

I don't need to be broken.

Whether I need it or not, I have been. There is a pause in the crop's steady rhythm, but I am still surprised when I feel the cock in my mouth. The ring gag and my bonds make it impossible for me to resist its penetration. My nose is clogged from my crying, and the cock makes it suddenly hard to breathe. I gag and try to turn away, and at the same time realize that it represents my salvation. While I'm sucking, while I'm serving it, the riding crop will stay still. If I can bring the cock to orgasm I will earn my relief from its sting. I know what's expected of me, what's required of me.

With suddenly renewed energy I bob my head up and down as much as the restraints will allow, eagerly fellating it. I run my tongue around the head, huge and swollen and salty, filling my mouth to overflowing. The ring gag denies me the use of my lips, but I know that the most erotic part of this encounter is not the touch of my flesh but my eager participation in my own humiliation, in my willing self-reduction to a sex object, and so I do my best to demonstrate that eagerness. The cock swells further, and I can feel that even the overstretching ring gag is a tight fit for it. I can taste the sweet-salt of precum on my tongue, feel its slippery texture oozing from the slit at the cockhead. It becomes my world, and even as I struggle to breathe around it, I want more, I want it forced all the way down my throat, I want to die impaled on it. I service it eagerly, desperate now to feel the splash of seminal fluid, no longer because his orgasm will save me further punishment but just because I want it, because I need to be fully complicit in the degradation of my essential self.

Degradation. It is hard to imagine a more humiliating position to be in, bound, stripped, my tits whipped, my cunt punished to the point of tears, and now forced to suck a total stranger's cock. I have no identity here, I'm just a fleshy masturbation aid, my value beginning and ending with my sexual openings. Nobody here cares about my first class degrees, about my carefully nourished career, about my wonderful, gentle husband. Nobody cares about anything except that I suck hard and long, and that I swallow when I'm done.

And oh, how I long to swallow, how I long to demonstrate that I am not just obedient, not just eager, that I am compelled, addicted, helpless before this cock. I need to prove that I am willing to do more, to go farther than anyone else he's ever been with, that I can take all he can give me and still beg for more, that I am worthy of being his chosen slut tonight. The cock grows stiffer, the head swelling to bursting tightness as I urgently tongue it in between thrusts. I should perhaps wonder about this man, but I don't. Whoever he is, he enjoys special status at this club. Whoever he is, Ninja Girl approves of him. Whoever he is, four women were lined up to undergo this initiation at his hands. These things are recommendation enough for me.

Is tonight a special night that I have somehow stumbled on, or does he do this every night? It doesn't matter. I hear him grunt, his thrusts coming more vigorously, gagging in their depth, and I work his cock harder, silently praying for him to anoint me with his white hot juice. And then suddenly he is, his hands pulling hard on my hair, his cock forcing itself to the back of my throat and beyond, swelling, exploding, jetting his sperm so deep, so forcefully that I don't even have the choice of not swallowing. His orgasm subsides, but he leaves his stiff swollen member in my mouth, and I diligently clean it with my tongue.

Finally he pulls out. "Good girl." His voice is deep and gravely, his breathing not fully recovered, and his words are more rewarding than orgasm. His still sticky cock nudges my face, the spermatic fluid still oozing from the tip leaving sticky trails on my cheeks. I feel heroic somehow, and I wish this moment could be televised so the whole world could see, so my husband especially could see. See me in this position with this man's sperm on my face and lips. I become aware of the wetness between my legs, and I realize that I've soaked myself to the knees. I'm such a slut.

Part Eight

Yeah you know me. You know everything about me. Not the trivialities like favourite music and taste in wine. You know what matters, you know what I like, you know what I am like. We've traveled this road so far together, honey, and through the journey you've learned who I am and how I am and the way I live. You know more about me now than family knows, more than my friends have learned in their whole lives. That's something special, honey. I've had women in my bed, women in my life who have never, ever seen this side of me, though some of them might have guessed. You have some of my most intimate secrets here, because I can't write this without letting you see the inner me, the secret side of myself.

Yeah, you know me. You even almost know my name. Yes, it's been changed here to protect the guilty, cleverly morphed just enough that someone won't suddenly learn more than they ever wanted to know. You don't *need* my name, though when you learn it you won't be surprised. What matters is, you know *me*, and I know you have a picture of me in your mind. Can you see me now, right there with you? Can you feel me, can you sense the warmth of my body, so close to yours? What do you call it when we're together? Making love? Fucking? It's both those things and more. I know how open it makes you feel, how vulnerable you are at that moment when I have you spread and wet and begging for it. I know how you yearn for it even as it scares you to be that exposed, not just your body, not just your cunt, but your mind, your soul. Do you have any idea what that does to me? Do you have any idea how your openness brings out my own?

Imagine me for a moment, right here on the other side of this page. Imagine me here with my mind focused on you. Picture every detail, my face, my expression, picture my shoulders, picture my waist, picture my legs, and oh yes, honey, picture the swelling bulge right there at my crotch. Imagine me imagining you. See me call you up in my mind's eye and realize how much I want you, you my perfect woman, you my one in a million, my one in ten million, my only one in all the universe.

Watch me shape you, one word at a time, line by line, every thought, every curve, every glance and smile. Imagine how long I've looked, how many women have come and gone to drive me to write this. Can you sense my story

Part Eight

in these words? You already know it, the mirror image of your own. I have a hunger, honey, I have a thirst, and you are my full course fantasy, my ideal woman made flesh and blood. Yeah, you know me. I'm the one who's been in your dreams since you first realized that boys might feel good. I'm the one who was there when everyone else thought you were asleep, when your fingers strayed down between your legs to explore the feelings that grew there. I'm the one in those dark and dangerous fantasies that you never quite revealed in those teenage games of truth or dare.

Yeah, you know me. I'm there in those comforting moments when you're by yourself but not alone. I'm there when you're out with friends with your eyes on the options that are good enough for them but not for you. We've come so close to meeting, time and time again. Remember when our eyes met, and the whole room vanished except you and me. You knew at that moment, you felt it in your bones. Remember when your friend took your attention and when you looked back I was gone? We missed that opportunity, honey. We missed it and we'll never get that time back, but the future is still ours.

Lay back, honey. Let me lie beside you. Undress for me, because you know I love the way you look in just your skin. Let me look at your breasts, smooth and firm and rounded and feminine, let me see your trim waist and the flare of your hips. Roll over for me, honey, let me be amazed at the shape of your taut ass. Has it recovered from your spanking yet? Let me run my hands down your body, and be amazed at the faces you present, good girl, bad girl, urban girl, nature girl, artist, professional, lover, friend.

Do you know what I love most about you? It's your curiosity, your thirst for knowledge. It's your clear thinking, the way you see right to the heart of a problem. It's your instinctive competitiveness, the way you never, ever want to be anything less than the very best. And more than that it's your playfulness, your lighthearted, unselfconscious ability to have fun, be silly, to laugh at yourself and with everyone around you.

Are you surprised again, honey? Did you think what I valued most was your body? Yeah, your body matters. Your body is built for sex, and sex is what it's about. If it weren't for sex you'd just live with your best friend and skip the complicated issues of male and female. If it weren't for sex you wouldn't put yourself through the heartache, if it weren't for sex you wouldn't be reading this book. Sex is primal, sex is power, sex is what makes the sparks fly, and anyone who says otherwise is denying reality. You have to have a good body to get with me, honey, it's the price of admission. Sex is the foundation, for what we're building here.

But it's only the foundation. Good bodies aren't hard to find. There are enough hot little sluts in the world willing to get their asses in the air for me to keep my cock wet for the rest of my life. Did I say willing? I meant eager. I meant fucking obsessed with the concept. And yeah, it's a trip to have some random hottie I met four minutes ago sink down on her knees with the sole objective of getting my cock inside her, but I need a little more than that. I need a lot more than that. I need a woman who can challenge me, who can surprise me, who's strong enough, smart enough to make it worth my while. I need that way more than firm tits and a tight ass, which isn't to say that I don't need those too. Good bodies aren't hard to find, but good minds are rare. Unique. Priceless.

So let me hold you, honey. Let me pull you close, pull you tight and inhale your scent. Let me run my fingers over the texture of your skin, let me learn the pattern of your body. Sex is the foundation, but intimacy is what's built on it, that special closeness. Do you have any idea how you rip me open, how you spill my soul across your bed? This isn't the game we started with honey, this is too true for that. The road has turned a corner, and now the journey begins for real. You open me when you open yourself, and I have no more choice to respond to you than you have to me. We're in free fall here, with nothing to do but hold on tight and pray for a soft landing. Let me hold you, honey, here in midair, in this dark and warm and timeless place, suspended in your mind. Let me hold you and feel your warmth, your touch, your soul. Let me cup your breast, lay my cheek on your belly, while you run your fingers through my hair. Can I trust you honey, really trust you? Do you want me, or just the fantasy I'm spinning here for you? And yes the fantasy is me, but it isn't all of me, and I need you to know all of me, want all of me, love all of me.

Yes love, I said it, that dangerous four letter word. I can't be with someone without loving them, some way, some how. I can't be with someone without giving them part of myself. Sex is about procreation, the closest commingling of two people that can ever be. DNA unwinding is the ultimate unzipping, the exposure of raw codons for the intimacy of crossover, the consummation of fertilization. Sexual bonding is no accident; it's built on the biological core of the act.

We call it love but you can't describe it, only experience it, and you know exactly what I mean. Surrender and possession, capture and release union and reunion. There's more truth in the final moment of climax than in all the words ever written. Love is a force of nature, *the* force of nature. Birds do it, bees do it, and yes honey, you and me do it. That has nothing to do with whether you want a baby or not, your body doesn't know about birth control, all it knows is how to respond to the presence of an alpha male. That's something too primal to think about, you just have to act.

Have I scared you, honey? Ruined your demon lover fantasy? Do you want to avoid emotion and intimacy and stay with primitive instinct - keep the image and lose the person behind it? The trick here is they aren't so far apart, love and lust, fantasy and reality. Not so far apart, but on opposite ends of the universe. I need all of you, and I need you to need all of me, rich or poor, sick

Part Eight

or healthy, everything I am. I need you deeply, not just the depths of your open and willing body but the very depths of your soul. I need it all. Can you give me that? Will you give me that? Because yes, honey, that's what I want, that's what I need.

Yeah, you know me honey, you know me better than anyone else and I am as open to you as I have ever been, as I have never been before. And I could seduce you right now, could slide you into the decision I want with the same fluid words that have kept you glued to these pages all this time. But I'm not going to, because I don't want you because I've seduced you, I don't want you because I've clouded your mind with desire. I want your decision, clear eyed and clear headed. I want you to choose, not have me choose for you. The door is right there in front of you, and you have to decide if you want to go through it, or turn away. Every door in the world is our door, and every time you have to make the choice to go through it.

So think it over, honey, take some time. Think about what we've had here and what we've done here and decide if you want more. You can see where this little adventure is going now and you know it's getting more and more real with every page you turn. It's for you to decide honey, yes or no, stop or go, carry on the journey or close the book and forget it ever happened. Go ahead and weigh it honey, don't cheat yourself, don't cheat me, by zipping on ahead. Make your decision a good one, because one way or the other there's no going back. Take your time, I'll wait on the next page, an hour or a day or forever. I'm patient that way.

Part Eight

And here you are honey, through the door, going down the road, and let me hug you and kiss you and tell you how glad I am to see you. Let me pick you up and spin you around and just be overjoyed at your presence. Let me put you down and lie down beside you and kiss you and hold you and cherish this moment. You and I. Us. Beautiful.

Bike Girl III

Kneeling, trussed, used, abused and degraded, a stranger's cock in my mouth, his sperm sticky on my face, it occurs to me to wonder where Ninja Girl has gone. Did she watch my subjugation? I find myself hoping that she has, that she enjoyed it, that it made her wet. I expect to find out soon, expect my ordeal to be over now that he's finished, but I'm wrong. They leave me there, hanging, sperm drying on my face, my juices drying on my thighs.

The arousal fades and leaves discomfort, in my knees, in my shoulder, in my back and most especially in my jaw, which has been hurting since it was first forced open by the cruel ring gag.

I can hear voices in the background, the man and, yes, it's Ninja Girl. I find some satisfaction in her presence. Their voices are casual, not quite loud enough for me to make out the words, and I imagine them with drinks in the hands, dispassionately contemplating my violated body as I hang there, on display for them. I am an object, and the discomfort of my position and the lingering pain in my tits and crotch combine to underscore the fact that my desires are simply irrelevant here. I shift position as much as I can to take the strain off my knees. I can take more strain off them if I transfer weight to the rope attached to the harness holding in the ring gag, but that forces the gag deeper into my mouth and makes the ache in my jaw excruciating. There's nothing I can do about the pain in my shoulders, or my wrists, or my ankles.

I need to urinate, badly, but I refuse to. I am not yet so fully degraded that I'll surrender control of my bladder. *Not yet.* It occurs to me that sooner or later even this threshold will be crossed, if that's what they want to happen they'll just leave me hanging until it does. It's no longer my decision whether I soil myself or not. I shudder at the realization. I wanted to be out of control and now I am. Despite the discomfort the thought is exciting.

At first it's exciting, but more time passes, and I drift into a strange place, talking to myself in my head about nothing, willing myself to get through the next hour, the next minute, the next ten seconds. I am dizzy, disoriented and the time seems unendurable. I was crazy to want this, crazy to volunteer for it, and I promise myself that if I ever get free I'll never go riding on the full moon nights again. *I promise, I promise, I promise.*

Bike Girl III

The pain won't go away and so I endure it, moment by moment. I'm still promising myself when fingers rub against my clit and out of nowhere my orgasm hits me with brutal, overwhelming force. I scream through the gag, and scream and scream and keep screaming as my body bucks hard against the restraints. My skin is on fire and my limbs are numb and the world goes red and then black. I have never had such a release in my life. I am dimly aware of hands on me, and I float away on a cloud of euphoria, as I'm lifted, as my tortured limbs are released, and at some point I drift off to sleep.

A long time later I wake up. Sunlight is streaming in the window. I'm in a strange bed, a soft one, beneath a thick, fluffy comforter. I squint against the brightness, find myself in a bedroom. I'm naked, but I always sleep naked and it occurs to me that perhaps I dreamed the entire night. I stretch, feel soreness in my joints beneath an overwhelming sense of completeness and satisfaction.

Did it really happen?

The events of last night seem distant and surreal, the woman whose memories fill my mind seems so unlike me. The bed is a canopy bed, and in a mirror over the dresser against the far wall I can see myself. My face is relaxed, calm, as after a good night's sleep. *Where am I?* It must all have been a dream, but then I move and my tender nipples rub painfully on the fabric of the comforter. I lift it and look down, see angry red lines still etched on my breasts, fading now to black and blue.

It happened.

I reach up to touch my face, feel the dried sperm still caked on my cheeks. Down between my legs, my clit is still throbbing and painfully sensitive when I reach down to touch it.

It really happened.

Lower still my thighs are crusted with my dried sex juices, messily mixed with fresh arousal still oozing from my overstimulated cunt. I feel a momentary revulsion, my calm satisfaction suddenly overturned.

It happened and I liked it, and I'm sick, sick, sick.

The dark fantasies of my moonlight rides are one thing, safely confined in my head, this was something else, this was real. Those fantasies weren't meant to be made real, shouldn't be made real, *couldn't* be made real. *And yet, Dear God, they have been*. They have come to life, and I am no longer an upwardly mobile professional woman, no longer the youngest senior partner in my firm, no longer the loyal wife and dutiful daughter. I have become... *what?* A whore? No not even a whore because I hadn't been paid. What kind of woman knelt to wait to perform oral sex on a stranger? The word 'slut' didn't cover it. What kind of woman allowed herself to be tied and whipped? A slave, perhaps? But even slaves don't enjoy it. The memory of that orgasm comes back to me and I shudder involuntarily. I have never responded like that, ever, not to my husband, not to anyone, not even to my bike.

Adrenaline suddenly spikes in my system. *It's morning. He'll be worried about me, he'll probably have called the police by now...* The door opens and Ninja Girl comes in with breakfast on a platter. The warm smell of eggs and oatmeal fills the room, and I realize I'm starving.

"I have to call..." I say.

"Your husband." she finishes. "I've already called him, he knows you're safe." I raise my eyebrows and she answers my unspoken question. "His number was in your phone." She sits down on the comforter beside me. It occurs to me that if my husband knows I'm safe he knows more than I do, although the pleasant surroundings and breakfast in bed don't seem nearly as dangerous as what I went through last night. Still, I don't know where I am, or who these people are.

"I'm to look after you," Ninja Girl says, plumping the pillow up so I can sit upright. I catch my own scent, dried sweat and sex, well ripened overnight. I need a bath, badly. She looks fresh scrubbed, clinically clean and I feel dirty beside her. With the comforter below my breasts she can see the welts on my breasts. She runs a finger gently over them, over the nipple, making me wince.

"You had a challenging night," she says, and aims a spoonful of warm oatmeal at my mouth, feeding me like a baby.

I dodge the spoon. "What did you tell him?"

"That I was a friend, that you'd stayed late in a club, and couldn't drive home, that I was taking care of you."

It was true enough, though I prayed she had omitted the deeper details. I nodded and she went on. "He's calling you in sick." She persisted with the spoon. The oatmeal was spicy with cinnamon and sweet with honey, mixed with thick cream, and heavenly. I hadn't realized how ravenous I am, and there is silence while she finishes feeding me. She'd brought fresh orange juice as well, and I drink that down while she holds the glass for me. It's odd to be treated like a child, but strangely comforting. I finish the eggs on my own.

"Do you want more?" Her eyes meet mine.

"More breakfast?"

"More everything." My heart started pounding and my breath caught in my throat. I ached everywhere, but the strongest ache was deep inside and what it ached for was exactly the *everything* she was offering. Just like last night, only this time I would know in advance what I was getting into. And this time, it wouldn't be just one night.

My mind spins at the concept, the conflicting desires her suggestion has aroused. "I don't... don't know..."

She nods. "The bathroom is there." She points to a door. "Your clothing is on the dresser, your bike is outside. You can go whenever you're ready. If you want more, go down the hall to the left, to the room at the end." She leans over to kiss my cheek. "You were beautiful. I want you to know that. You were perfect."

She smiles and leaves, and I stretch and get up and go to the window to look out into a lovely, mature garden. The house is old, with high, molded ceilings and high, wide windows. I look down at my welted breasts. I would have to wear a nightgown to bed for a week, stop my husband from seeing me until the bruises faded, but that wouldn't be difficult. Last night had been... what? *An adventure, nothing more.* It had been fantasy explored, intensity discovered, opportunity seized, but it wasn't real life. I run my fingers over the red weals. They're already fading, and I find I don't want them to. They are badges of honour, proof that I've sustained my ordeal. I touch my sperm encrusted cheek again, remembering how I'd felt when my master came on my face. *My master.* I shook my head. That man, whoever he was, was certainly masterful, but he wasn't my master. My storybook life was waiting back in my home, with my husband, with my firm, with my family, and it was time to reclaim it.

I turn from the window and go into the bathroom to find a huge, old fashioned tub with an overhead shower, fresh towels, soap and bath salts, everything sparkling and clean. I turn on the shower, run it steaming hot and get in, only to find the shower jets painful on my tenderized skin. I flip the valve to run the bath instead, add bath salts and ease myself into the heat. It feels wonderful, languid and relaxing, and I scrub myself clean of sweat and sex while I let the tub run full, then relax and let the heat soothe the remaining aches of last night's adventure. I had been beautiful, she said. *Perfect.* My competitive instinct smiles a little smile of smug satisfaction. I had been dirtier, needier, sluttier than any of the others, those who hadn't been chosen, and I had gone on to prove the wisdom of their choice. It's a character flaw that drives me to be the best at everything, even things that it isn't good to be the best at.

Real life. I climb out of the tub and towel off, feeling reborn. As she has promised my leathers are folded neatly on top of the dresser, my helmet on top of them, riding boots neatly arranged on the floor. I touch them, feeling the texture of my heavy second skin. I become a different person when I put them on, they are the key to my full-moon ovulation transformation. This time I became a different person when I took them off – *when they were taken off me* – and now they seem like a caterpillar's cocoon, shed to reveal a butterfly. I smile to myself again.

Yes it was worth it. I had changed, learned things about myself and that was always a good thing, even if I never repeated the experiment. I pick up the pants and check the crotch, and find they've been cleaned, the sticky evidence of my long arousal now gone. Tentatively I bring them to my nose, sniff gently, and catch just a hint of my own scent, still clinging there despite the cleaner's best efforts. As with me the change is invisible, but indelible. I dress, pull on my boots, pick up my helmet and go out. I'm in a wide carpeted hall opposite a railing. On the floor below is a beautiful entryway. The stairs down are to my right. I can see my beloved Harley, parked in the driveway through the large windows on the lower floor. I glance left. At the end of the hall is a pair of paneled double doors.

If you want more, go to the room at the end of the hall. There's no-one around. I shake my head. *Time to go.* Down the stairs and out the door to my bike, my home, my husband, my life. Time to recover who I was, who I am, who I am supposed to be. Time to put this all behind me, in that secret store of memory, a test faced, passed, and put behind.

And yet...

I hesitate, look to the paneled double doors, look back to my bike. *What could be behind them?* A different life, a different me, an unknown future. *What could be waiting for me there?* I go down the hall to the doors, not because I've changed my mind about staying, but out of curiosity. I don't know what I expect to find, implements of bondage and punishment most likely, perhaps the man who had used me last night. I'm overcome with the sudden urge to look him in the eye, to let him know the change he has wrought, and to let him know that still, I remain myself, even more myself than I was before we met. I push gently. The doors are heavy, and silent on their hinges, and what I find behind them is a library, three walls lined with close-packed bookshelves, the fourth with various pieces of art, paintings, little sculptures, a pair of crossed swords that look very old. There is a wide mahogany desk in front of a heavy, red leather chair in the center of the room, and nothing more. Not even a riding crop. The place smells of books.

I feel vague disappointment, I'd been hoping for something more thrilling. I shrug, turn to go, then turn back. It was the desk that drew me in. It was the desk, heavy, shiny, polished, black, that triggered something in my brain, something I couldn't even begin to resist. I want what it has, I need it, and so with trembling fingers, unable to think, I undress, leaving everything in a tangled pile. I walk over to the end of the desk and bend over it, spreading my legs wide, exposing my cunt, exposing all of me. He will bring the riding crop when he comes, I know that in my heart. My clit throbs in anticipation.

Part Nine

Bike Girl, thrice purified, first with her bike, then with the riding crop, the last time with her bath. She's taken the fork in the road, chosen to come through the door. That's your story too, honey, down our road, through our door, coming to me for the purification, the concentration, the liberation of your own secret self. Now it's your bath time, honey. Remember that nice story I wrote about the bath, way back at the beginning of our journey? Time to make it real. You need to do this in the evening, right before bedtime. And you need to have nice soap, bath salts, fresh new razor, bath scrub, candles and a glass of wine. Bring your fluffiest towels, have them ready so they'll be nice and warm and cozy for when you're done. Make sure you use the washroom before you begin, honey. We don't need you getting distracted halfway through. Disconnect the phone, close the door behind you. Close the door and lock it, because this time is just for me and you. Make sure your bed is made up nice and fresh, because you're going straight there afterwards. Get your coziest PJs out, neatly folded on your pillow. Get it all ready and come back tonight.

Part Nine

Welcome back, bath girl, time to start. Into the bathroom and run the tub as hot as it will go, steaming, scalding, way too hot to get into, trust me now. Put in the bubbles or the salt or whatever girly bath stuff it is you have. While it's filling pour the wine and set it down, get your nice fluffy towels. Get your scrubber and your razor and soap and shampoo and light the candles. This is going to be you and me alone and it's going to be so nice, honey. We're going to make you a new woman, head to toe. And you *are* a new woman, aren't you, honey, changed so much since we started this journey. You're *my* woman now, my good girl.

Candles lit now, then get undressed, and turn off the water when the tub is full. Yes I know it's far too hot to get in yet, so you're going to have to wait a little while. And the way I want you to wait is with your legs apart and straight, bent over at the waist with your hands on the edge of the bathtub. A little awkward, yes, a little uncomfortable, but very, very necessary, to put you in the proper mindset for getting your bath.

Yes, honey. I want you feeling very pliant and submissive before you get in, and this is the position to achieve that. You're going to wait there until that steaming water cools to the right temperature, and then you're going to ease yourself in. And while you're waiting you can think about anything you like, although if you chose to think of the inherent vulnerability of your position here, if the thoughts that go through your mind are about having me stand beside you, behind you, having me caress you, having me squeeze your delightfully hanging breasts, having me tweak your already aroused nipples, having me probe your exposed and helpless openings while you wait, that is perfectly fine with me.

So think your thoughts, honey, and enjoy your time in this position, and when the water is right, just right, turn the page.

Part Nine

And now you're going to get in the tub, and the trick here is that while the water isn't quite scalding anymore, it's still as hot as you can stand it, isn't it? You didn't want to wait face down and ass up any longer than you had to, so now you're in and it's hot, hot, *hot*. Feel the heat soak into your bones, and just lie back and relax for a long, slow minute. Take your time, feel your muscles start to relax, feel the heat and the moisture wash away the tension. Drink your wine and just let your mind float. Let it float away, just read the page while I say, float away, float away, float away, and your mind is floating away, everything is peaceful and dreamy and quiet and warm and you're just floating away on a nice warm cloud. Baths are good for that, baths are beautiful for that, baths restore and refresh and wash everything bad away.

Breathe in and breathe out and just keep floating, and notice how good it feels to just surrender for a little while. We're going to cleanse not just your body but your mind, clean you completely, and so just breathe in and breathe out and let yourself float, let yourself be free and you might choose to think of a warm beach with the waves lapping and the gentle wind blowing, and the heat is soothing your muscles and your soul at the same time. And when you're ready, honey, when you're just as smooth and soothed as soothed can be, just inhale one more time, slow and deep, and hold it, and let yourself slip under water, and stay there for a little while, and when you're ready again, just come back up.

Beautiful. This is immersion and rebirth, the return to the womb, and you are so very much mine right here and right now. And now we're going to start washing, and it's going to be me washing you, that's the way it's going to be. Ready? We'll start with the right hand washing the left arm, soap on, scrub it down, nice brisk motions, get every last inch, do it firmly, do it thoroughly, soap off. Now switch, left washes right, the same as before. Isn't that nice, isn't that easy?

And so now we're going to wash your face, scrub it thoroughly, forehead and cheeks and chin, each side of your nose, and your eyes and your ears. Rinse it once, rinse it twice, and move on to your graceful neck, feel your pulse in your throat as you clean around, and down over your collarbones. Do your shoulders, left and right, scrub them hard. Do each breast, and your nipples are so very sensitive under the rough scrubber, but do them as thoroughly as the rest. Do your armpits, and don't worry about shaving, we'll get to that later. Reach back for your back, left and right, do it well, and already you're feeling cleaner, feeling fresher. Do your stomach and sides, and make sure you get your belly button.

Isn't this nice, honey? Isn't this warm and intimate? Do you know how wonderful it is for me to give you a bath, to treat you like my very own special girl, to share this time? I love to be intimate with you, even more than I love to be sexual with you, though sexuality is intimate of course, and intimacy is sexy.

The Secret Journey

Still there is a difference, and right now is so very intimate, so very close, and I just want to climb in there with you. I'm not going to though, not this time, because this is my time to look after you, and your time to be looked after.

So let me keep scrubbing, honey, down to your hips and your thighs and your vulva. That's right, honey. Raise a leg so I can get in between, every inch must be clean. And the scrubber is rougher on your clit than it was on your nipples, and you have to spread those pretty lips to get every last crevice, and down lower over your tight little anus, and raise both legs to get each buttock, left and right, full and firm, scrubbed hard until they blush pink. Beautiful.

Remember last time your ass blushed for me? Remember the stinging smacks, how you wiggled and struggled but had to take each one. This time is much nicer, isn't it? Much more tender, much more gentle, and yet still a reminder of how you felt that time. The memory brings back those feelings, and mixes them up with what you're feeling now, all warm and clean and relaxed. The truth is you've been cleansed both times, purified as Bike Girl was. The truth is you need each side, up and down, hard and soft, yin and yang, you and me. And now your thighs, scrubbed down, top and bottom and all around, special attention to the back of the knee. Calves scrubbed just the same, and then each foot, top and bottom, and your ankles, and each little toe. Don't forget to do in between.

Clean now, top to toe, but not done yet. Time for the razor now. Armpits first, do them carefully, do them smooth. I like a girl's armpits clean, clean. Do left and do right, and when they're done check them, run a hand over to make sure there's no stubble. Clean up any you find, and then we're done. Legs next, long, smooth strokes. Do you wax? Today you're shaving. Take it slow, do them justice. Shaving is like stripping, and a freshly stripped woman is extra naked, extra sexy.

And you know what's coming next, don't you? You know I'm going to have you do your pussy too. You know you're going to come out of this bath as naked as the day you were born. And you know I like this honey, but not for the reason you think. I do like smooth legs and smooth armpits, but I also like to know I'm with a woman, a mature, ripe and fertile woman. I don't want the illusion that I'm with a prepubescent girl, not where it counts.

And so go ahead, honey. Start on your pubic hair. Do you do this as a part of your routine, is it just a matter of cleaning up the stubble? Or do you never shave your pussy at all? Do you have to take your time on it, go slowly and carefully? I would like to know my dear, as much as I'm sure you would like to know why it is I'm shaving you, even though I prefer women *au naturale* between the legs. So I'll tell you what, you shave, take your time, and I will explain while you do. It's very simple really, and it has nothing to do with what I like, or what you like. It has everything to do with the way this relationship works, which is that I get to be in charge, I get to make the decisions on the

Part Nine

most intimate topics imaginable, like whether you shave your pubic hair or not. What matters is not which way I prefer it, what matters is you make a physical change to demonstrate that yes, you agree, I get to make the decisions.

Say "Yes," for me honey. "Yes."

"Yes sir, you get to decide."

And keep shaving. Get it all, get it smooth, good girl.

So because of the way this is working, with so much time between my *now* and yours, I can't know whether you normally go around shorn or unshorn, not now, not yet. And so the only way to guarantee that you're going to make a change is to start with you shaved, and then have you grow it back in. That way you make a change for sure, and that way I get to have you the way I want you, when the change is finally done.

And you do know how very much I want to have you, don't you honey? Very much, indeed.

Au naturale. Today you're shaving for me, after today you won't ever shave again. And the whole time that it's all growing back, every day of longer and longer hair, you'll be reminded of the reason you're going through the exercise, which is because I want you to and for no other reason. You'll be reminded when you dress in the morning, and when you strip at night. You'll be reminded when you take a shower, and especially when you take a bath. You'll be reminded every time it occurs to you to think of it, and it will occur to you to think about it often, because you're going to find yourself even more obsessed with this, obsessed with me, than you have ever been before.

And that's saying a lot, isn't it honey. Because you and I both know how your thoughts turn to me at the most unusual times. We both know the flood of arousal that hits you at random moments in the middle of the day, whenever you look at a door, our door, whenever you go stand on the road that connects us. Those things make you think of our journey, and they make you wonder *what is he doing now? Now?*

But that's for tomorrow, that obsession, and this is tonight, this is bath time, intimate time, not sex time. And so once you're done shaving, once your pussy is clean and smooth, we're going to carry on with bath time. Water out, shower on, time to rinse, starting with your hair. First rinse just takes off what's left of the soap, face and neck and arms. Body, front and back, and between your buttocks, and down each leg. Are you having trouble reading this and showering at the same time? I'm smiling as I think of you doing it, slightly silly, isn't it? But fun, very fun, and only you and I will know. So now we're going to wash your lovely tresses. Head under the shower again, shampoo in and scrub it hard, squeeze the suds through, get them everywhere, and then rinse, rinse it so well, and do it again, with half as much shampoo this time. That's the key to rinse and repeat, using half as much the second time. Squeeze it through again, and I'm sure your fingers and toes are getting wrinkled by now. That's okay, honey, because we're almost done, though we'd both like this to last forever.

Second rinse now, for all of you, water on full, notch up the heat, and go over every last part of you, slowly, slowly, getting all the places soap can stick. Get your hair soaked, get behind your ears. Do the underside of your breasts, and it's alright if you jump as the spray comes across your nipples. Get your belly and back, and get up between the cheeks of your ass, and your pussy, and all around. Get between each finger, and get between each toe, and smile because you're done at last, spic and span.

Water off and out of the bath and into the first warm, fluffy towel. Dry off your body, face, left arm, right arm, back, front, left leg, right leg, both feet all ten toes, and both hands, and then do your hair. Wrap the towel around your hair when you're done, wrap the second towel around you, and off to your bed.

And then - towels off, PJs on. Slide yourself down between the sheets, and feel me tucking you in, making sure you're as snug and safe as you are pink and clean. Feel me hug you, big and easy. Feel me kiss you on the cheek, and you can smile and giggle and get another kiss, just for being so cute, so special, so mine. Feel me look at you with warmth and tenderness, feel the specialness of *now*, feel the intimacy of this moment that is yours and mine and no-one else's.

And snuggle down to sleep tight, and know that I am watching over you.

Dance Girl

Club time. I love the music, that dark pounding beat that turns on the heat, sets up the groove, drives my body to move. I love the scene, lights and lasers, smoke and mirrors, hot boys and hotter girls, flash passion on the floor with some random Romeo. It pumps my mind to bump and grind, and what gets me wet isn't the men but my power over them. Hook him in, tease him hard, rub him with my bouncing body, spin around, arch my back and feel my victory, hard through his jeans against my ass, then spin again, back into the circled girl-twirl, seal him out, ignore him while his lust goes limp.

I watch him leave, then ride the dance trance, grinding chicks until I need another power fix. I'm a sex vixen vampire, out all night stealing men's souls, then home at dawn to crash behind closed curtains for the day. Sunday's sunlight sears me. More to say the day's mundane demands suck my spirit dry. Monday morning strikes like lightning and I rise up from the slab, head into the lab. I slip on my dark glasses, show up for my classes but that woman isn't me. She's differential undead, a female form phantasm, with curves unintegrated, heated under constant pressure, and in thermodynamic equilibrium with Hell. Physics resonates but class work is nothing but viscous drag.

Friday freedom, dance trance. It's a six hour orgasm and the floor is packed with sweat and sex. I'm here to claim what's mine, and I measure my night by the boys I score, though I've always lost track by twelve. I dress in class-trash, tight little slut-skirt and fuck-me-now boots, show enough to make them want me, style enough to be out of their league. Dance trance. They want to fuck me but I'm a show-girl not a go-girl, married to the music and ever faithful to the beat. I get all I need in their desire, and ride the rhythm all night long. Do it, do it hard, play it loud, pound it in me, slam me with ten thousand watts root-mean-square. I have my place, right where the big bass driver makes the very air shake.

Pump it up, pump it out, pump it in me. I spin up and do the splits on the speaker's top, feel the bass beat my body right where I need it most and shudder through the climax, jerking to the music. In that instant every man's fantasy is that I'm coming right in front of them, little knowing that I really am. Spin back down before I'm caught, I'm not allowed to do it, I just need to. Fuck them all,

Dance Girl

and every cock is hard as rock, as I rock hard for them, even if it's too dark to see the dirtier details of my depraved display.

Fuck yes, I'm a dirty girl for someone still a virgin. I lock eyes with uber-jock, hard muscle ready to tussle, a tall-lean-square double-dare. I let him scope me, want to grope me, let him dance over, then slide my hands down his arms, feel his strength. He moves well, and I can tell his body will know what to do. I let him kiss me so I know he'll miss me, and my entire body is electrified as the high-voltage sparks fly. I turn around and give him the bump-and-grind, arch my back. I look over my shoulder, see his face, know that he'd fuck me on the floor, if he could, if I would. I give it to him until he's ready to blow and then I go, spin-spin back into the girl-twirl, my bass-bouncing chastity belt. I'm so energized I double up the beat, moving to the centre so he can't follow, moving too fast for him if he did. He tries to get in for more of my sin, but he fails to penetrate, leaves the tease in defeat and I score another notch for me. The light show flickers in my eyes, blurring out the world as the beat pounds my brain. *Take that, my leaving, lusting, love loser.* I'm the hottest slut in the room and I know it.

Dance trance, change tracks. I jump back to the fundamental frequency, move my body, let the lights streak as the world spins. The music shifts and I drop into rhythm with this gorgeous girl. She's just my height, just my build but light to my darkness with deep blue eyes and pure blonde hair. We phase-lock, push and pull, put on a private semi-sex show. She spins me around and we grind together, her snatch against my ass as hot as any denim-caged cock. This is my power, this is my moment, this gets the eyes back on my body where they belong, and I work her like a stripper on the pole. Every woman in here is dressed to kill and moves to thrill, but the girl-girl double play trumps them all.

Dance trance. I scan the hungry eyes, then close my own and let my play-partner have her way with me, hands on my waist, setting the rhythm, setting the motion. She spins me around, face to face and our breasts collide, rigid nipples score scorching lines over soft and supple skin. We're dancing dirty, and I let her go farther than I'd ever let a man, touching me, leading me through sinuosities guaranteed to pull in cocks like compass needles seeking north. I see us centred in a sacrificial circle, as the rigid, thrusting rods spurt sperm on the floor in ritual supplication to their sex goddess twins.

Dance trance, change tracks. She's a fine find, my anonymous Amazon, she knows how to work the crowd, how to work me, and she works me good. She spins me again, takes the lead with casual ease, her hands sliding over my curves with firm assurance. I spot my next tease-target, a leather-jacket bad boy, truck driver or hard rider, and either way he's dangerous goods with a long, wide load. I catch his eye and glance away, lure him in with his lust. He dances over, looking for the opening I'm about to give him and I let the moment build while I soak up the rush. A split-beat later I spin to let him in, but

The Secret Journey

my Amazon's hands keep me turning, past him and into her and then we're locked, eye to eye in a tit-tit collision, and I can feel her nipples hard on mine. She shakes her head, a tiny motion, telling me that he's out of bounds, and my world turns upside down.

Boys are toys and the way to win the girl-game is to collect the set, but Amazon is playing by different rules. She holds my gaze and I descend into the haze of her female sweat-scent. Her hands are on my body, moving me where she wants me to go. The world slows down. I close my eyes, let her do what she feels, and I can't believe it's really happening. The music fades to a distant roar and suddenly I'm on the half beat, the quarter beat, dephased from the rhythm and we're slow dancing, tight, tight, tight. I can't think, can barely breathe but my body knows what it wants, and my belly tenses, my pussy swells, ready for her to do whatever she likes.

Dance trance, change tracks. It's different now, not about the beat but the bubble that encases us, her warm form sliding against my skin, her scent and my own filling my world, my mind, my everything. I tremble because I'm terrified, my anti-slut secret is I've only ever kissed a boy, never even kissed a girl but I know it's going to happen now. I want to run and can't, I'm paralyzed, my vampire-vixen power drained like she's spiked a silver stake through my heart. Her hand slides up from the small of my back, up to my shoulders, up to my neck and I haven't got the strength to escape, and then she's doing it. She kisses me as if she has all the time in the world, slowly, softly, not even parting my lips. They part on their own and then she's exploring me and I can feel myself dissolve, all the power of my sexuality, extracted dance-erotic from a thousand-thousand men, she drains it out of me and into her.

I'm so weak I can barely stand and she's holding me up, still moving me, seducing me, and it happens all at once, no warning, my cunt clenching hard in sync with the beat, my climax and my first surrender. She captures my gasp with her lips and I have no memory at all of how we got to the bathroom stall. What I recall, what's seared into my brain is the pleasure and pain, and the sight of her sticky-slick slit. She sits splayed on the seat while I kneel on the floor, dirty knees as I strive to please. What's scorched into my memory is her touch, her scent, her musk-salt sex, enveloping me as I lap my tongue against her stiff-swollen clit, to prove to her that I am hers. I took it for her, took it all as her stickiness smeared my face, put me in my place, marked me as her territory. She held my hair, no longer gentle as she had danced. She was rough, because she could be rough. She had captured me and I was hers to use or abuse, and when she came she pulled so hard it hurt.

I didn't care. I wanted her to hurt me, I needed it so I could show how far she could go. I wanted her to love me and whip me and feed me and fuck me. I wanted her to hold me, punish me, tease me, please me, dress me and undress me, tell me I was a good girl and a bad girl but most of all *her* girl. She made me crave to be her slave, to crawl for her, beg for her, lick her boots, her cunt, her tits, her everything, and everywhere. I needed to take it all, have her give me more. And she did it and she still does it and my world is complete living at her feet.

Dance trance, change tracks, the music is different but the rhythm remains the same.

Part Ten

Class-trash is the way dance-girl dressed, when she wanted the attention on her. Class-trash is how I'm going to dress you, honey, for this next little step on our journey. This one is full-frontal audience participation, honey. It's going to take all day, so plan a day to spend with me, and come back that morning. I want you dressed in your class-trash best, and by that I mean your sluttiest little skirt and your most enticing stockings and your best come-fuck-me pumps. I want a tight little top so flimsy your nipples might tear holes in it. Skirt and top, stockings and shoes and that's all. You'll notice a complete absence of underwear on that list. No bra, no panties, you don't need them for this one. I want hooker-red on your lips, and no other makeup. I want you looking like a trashy street slut crossed with a high-priced whore. Do it for me honey, spend some time on it, make it good because you know you want to. Set up your best dance-beat music, and bring your digital camera. And honey? When you come make sure you lock our door behind you, and disconnect the phone.

I'll be seeing you soon.

Part Ten

Okay honey, now it's just you and me, alone and private. And now that you're dressed the part, I want you to take a good, long look in the mirror. Check out your tits, rub the nipples stiff so they stick through the fabric and feel my hands on them, grabbing them hard, mauling them like you were some cheap slut picked up in a sleazy dance bar. Check out your lips, vamped up with that fuck-me-now lipstick, and imagine how they'll look wrapped around my cock. Check out your ass, check out your legs in those heels. You're a slut here, honey, nothing more and nothing less. Now go set up the camera, set up the timer, set it up for video if you can, set up the lights and background. Now music *on*, and move to the beat. Don't just look the part, feel it, live it, *be* it.

I want you posing, sexy poses, revealing poses, slutty poses. I want you to vamp it right up, get into it, like a whore trying to raise her selling price. I want private poses, just for me, skirt-up poses, tits-out poses. I want you to move your body to the rhythm, get into it, do the slut-strut with a roll to your hips, work your body, put yourself on display. Strip to the music. Go on, move it honey, I want you to prance like the dirtiest girl at the dance. We're going to strip the veneer here, honey. No more nice girl, professional girl, none of that. I want you to be the total, utter street slut and nothing else. You're going to be my own personal pornstar, so get clicking, shoot yourself in the mirror if you have to, I don't care about artistic merit, I care about hot shots - tits, cunt and ass. Don't be shy, honey, the time for shyness with you and me is long, long past. Are you ready for your close-up? Do it, do it now.

Click, click, click, the camera loves you because, my God, you're such a hot little bitch. *Fuck yes, work it slut.* Come on, part your lips and pout sexy for me, make those big, big, bedroom eyes. Come on, part your legs and pout again, show me how trashy you can get. This excites your bad girl side, I know it does. Let's see how you look with one leg up so I can see up your skirt. Let's see how you look bent right over with your legs apart and your cunt exposed. I want to watch you give head to a banana, I want to see you lick ice cream from a bowl. Click, click, click. Now let's see how you look masturbating, peeling back the hood of your clit. Let's see how you look with your sticky fingers spreading your sticky pussy, and sliding inside. Go on, do it, and then lick them clean. Use your imagination, honey, and burn those images into your dirty little mind. Work it like a stripper, honey. Make it good, make it very good. Show me just how depraved you can be.

That's my bad girl, keep the shutter clicking in your very first porno photoshoot. It takes twenty frames to get one money shot, so take lots. I want to see everything. Play dress-up for me, I want you naked in boots, jerking off in bra and panties. I want everything from trashy-but-innocent to naughty teasing to dirty-dancing eager slut. I want you from every angle, every pose, every position. Keep your cunt open for it honey, keep your nipples stiff, keep your clit hard. Make it good, take your time. Come back when you're so hot you could scream, honey, but make sure it's at least an hour. I want you good and hot, and I want you to know just how far you'll go. Click, click, click. Go do your photo shoot, honey, and come back when you're mine in digital reality.

Part Ten

Welcome back, pornstar girl, how do you feel now? Hot and sexy, slutty, dirty, and oh, so turned on by this little adventure in private exhibitionism. It's a rush, honey, so ride it. I know you get wet doing it, and what I love is the way you get sexier when you get hot, how the juicing of your pussy shows up in your eyes, in your face. What I love is how the pose becomes reality as you arch your back and present your ass. What I love is how the desire to tease becomes the need to fuck as you flip your skirt up, and slowly expose more and more of your tits. I love how you twist your body to show it off. You're sending out a message here, and it's nothing more or less than "I'm hot and easy, come and fuck me." You're looking for that perfect pose that screams it out.

"I'm hot and easy, come fuck me."

Say it, honey. "I'm hot and easy, come fuck me."

"I'm hot and easy, cheap and sleazy, come fuck me like the whore I am." Say it, show it. Do we need more pictures, honey? Not enough there yet? Then get more for me, you know what I need from you.

Fuck, you're such a slut for me, my cock is so hard for you. And what I want you to do now is go through every image, every pose and look at yourself the way I look at you, raw, exposed, inviting, inciting, pure sex, and all woman. Concentrate on the swell of your tits and the curve of your ass and the glistening slit of your cunt. Concentrate on the shine in your eyes, look at the expression on the face of this girl who is you, this woman exposing herself for me. Look at the way she works her body, works her look, look at the way she's dressed for display. Think about what she's telling her audience. "I'm hot and easy, come and fuck me."

Go ahead and say it, honey. "I'm hot and easy, come and fuck me. Come fuck me, please. Please, please, please, come fuck me, *please!*"

Go through the pictures honey, and beg for it frame by frame. Beg with your voice, the way you beg with your body. Look at that dirty little slut in the digital mirror, uninhibited, wanton, sex personified, depravity purified. Tell that girl what you think of her, how how she is, how dirty she is. Tell her what a slut she is, what a horny little bitch. Tell her out loud, you know I like to hear you say it. If you can't say the words, you can't have the experience, so tell her very clearly exactly what you think. And spread those legs as you read this honey, as you look at your dirty-whore pornstar pics. Spread those legs and spread that sticky cunt wide for me. She needs to be fucked, honey, that dirty girl you are in the camera's eye is there to be fucked and nothing more. She needs it so bad. And there's one more thing you're going to do with this honey, now that you've chosen your perfect slut-wear, now that your body is trembling in sexual need. Finish going through your pictures, and I'll tell you when you turn the page.

Part Ten

Hot bitch, slutty bitch – done with your dirty pics, ready for your assignment now? It's easy. I want you to go shopping, go downtown, dressed just like this.

And I can hear the screech of your mental tires as you hit that corner. *What did he say?* You didn't expect that, did you, honey? Yeah, I'm sending you out in public. Does that scare you? Does that excite you? Yes it's another one of my little tests, designed to strip away the lesser women who've come into my world by mistake. Here's where the rubber meets the road, honey. Here's where we learn what you're made of. You're going out in your trashiest outfit, and you're going shopping for something even sluttier, while the men look with lust and the women stare with envy. Strut it, work it, tease the boys and taunt the girls. You're going to get hit on, but no giving out your number, that's against the rules, honey. You're out there to show, not to go. Are you brave enough to do this? We're about to find out.

Oh, and honey, while you're out, can you pick something up for me? Good girl. Just drop by the hardware store and pick up some rope, get white nylon twist, one quarter inch diameter. Get four pieces, one twelve yards long, the others twelve feet. Thanks, honey. I knew that I could count on you. Turn the page when you're back.

Part Ten

Welcome back, honey. How was your slut-strut? Did you feel the eyes on you, when you bought even trashier clothes. Did all those men want you while you displayed yourself like a shameless whore? You *know* what they were thinking when you bought that rope in the hardware store. And you know what I was thinking when I told you to get it. Yah, honey, I want you tied up, cunt up and begging for my cock, and yes, honey, that's exactly what I'm going to get. You know about rope and riding crops, honey. That's why you're here. You know about domination and submission, you've read stories, you've seen pictures, maybe you've even played games with a boyfriend or two. I've already taught you that pain can be pleasure, now you're going to learn that confinement can be freedom.

You're going to give yourself up to me, honey. You're going to give me everything. I know it and you know it, and we both want it, and the proof of that for me is the reality that you're reading this, and the proof of that for you is the fact that you've got the rope. You knew exactly what it was for the moment I mentioned it, and the knowledge has been wetting your cunt ever since. Hasn't it, you dirty little bondage slut?

You don't have to answer, honey, we both know the answer. So just pick up those ropes, feel them, explore the texture. Wrap them around your wrists and tug. You're going to be bound for me today, bound and helpless and completely mine. That thought sends a thrill through your clit, honey. That thought makes your pussy wet and your nipples tingle and your breath come short. Remember your earliest hazy dreams, bad girl dreams that were secret and steamy for reasons you didn't quite understand. Remember how exciting it was to imagine being captured by pirates, tied up in cops and robbers, caught and held in all sorts of ways. Remember hot defiance overlying those deeper feelings, being *taken*, taken past your defences, taken away from yourself. That was the start, honey. And now, here we are.

There's an art to erotic rope work, honey, the Japanese call it shibari and you're about to experience its intricacies. Don't hurry this one, take your time, make sure you do it right. Time to double-check, make sure the stove is off, make sure the phone is disconnected, make sure our door is closed and locked, we don't want any interruptions, honey. And when we do start we're going to start with the basics. This is shibari karada and the internet is your friend in learning, just make sure you get the right version, body-bound only. Start with the long rope. Drape it across your shoulders, the same as a shawl, one end hanging down over each breast, equal lengths on each side. Gather the two strands together, like you were going to tie a tie. Now you've got the two ends together, hanging down between your breasts. Hold them together like one rope, and put in a single-loop knot to sit right above your pretty tits. You don't need girl-scout skills here, honey, just make a loop and pass the free ends through.

Now you should have a loop around your neck with the free ends hanging free, just like a big, loose necktie. Simple. Are you're getting aroused at this? You will. I know you're anxious honey, anxious for this to go to its natural conclusion, anxious to feel restrained, immobilized, and mine.

The second knot goes between your breasts, a third below them, The fourth on your belly button, and the last one goes right at your clit. Take the free ends, run them between your legs, up the crack of your ass, up your back and through the loop at the back of your neck. Snug them up, feel them tighten, feel that last knot right up between your pussy lips, right where it's going to remind you what's happening. Take one free end, bring it around beneath your armpit, thread it through the space between the first two knots. Take it back behind your back and around to the other side, thread it through the space between the second knot and the third. Feel how that starts to present your tits. You see how it's working now, don't you honey? We're lacing you up tight, tight, tight. Now back around behind again, and around to thread between the third knot and the fourth. One more time, back around again and through above the knot at your clit, and tie it there. You're half-wrapped now, honey. Do the mirror image on the other side, top to bottom. Snug the rope tight and tie the ends off, my tight-bound little slave girl. It's tighter on your pussy now, that hard little knot putting your clit in its place. Karada is the rope dress, and here you're bound even when you're free. Try moving, feel how it tightens, how it restricts your movements, how the rope controls you with its very presence. You can wear this out beneath your dress and nobody would ever know. Nobody except you, and me.

Feel how it makes your cunt wet. Have you ever felt like this before, honey, bound and free at the very same time. And it's going to get better. Take a second length of rope, twelve feet long, then sit down on the floor, and you'll feel that clitoral knot remind you that it's there. Put your ankles together. Fold the rope double, pass the loop around your ankles and thread the free ends through it. Snug it tight and start wrapping, around and around, until you've got just two feet left. Then you're going to pass the rope down between your calves from in front, and then up between your feet from behind, wrapping the rope around the coils around your ankles. Do that once more, then the free ends go left and right around your ankles and get tied off in front. Snug but not too tight, honey. Don't cut off the circulation, that's a bad thing. There's a skill to this, learn it well.

Take the third length of rope and do the same thing above your knees. How are you feeling now, honey? Restrained. Vulnerable. Mine.

Fourth rope. You're sitting on the floor with your knees drawn up in front of you. Do the same thing at your wrists that you've done with your ankles. Save three feet for the cross wrapping part, and thread the free ends through the

Part Ten

rope at your knees, anywhere, it doesn't matter where. Do a few passes around and around. You won't be able to tie it off if you've done everything right, you won't have enough movement in your wrists. That doesn't matter honey, because it's the feeling of restraint that counts, and that's what you're getting from this.

I can do anything to you when you're like this, just pick you up and put you in position, to whip you, fuck you, or simply leave you there, decorative and available. You're my tied up little bondage slut now, honey. You're going to stay this way for exactly as long as I want you to. So we'll start out with an hour. It's going to get uncomfortable, and it might get boring, but what's important, honey is that you're mine, all mine, more mine than you have ever been. You'll feel that, deep inside you. You'll be wet by the end of it, aroused in a way you never thought possible. And when the hour is up you can undo your hands but nothing else, and you can rub your eager fingers over and under and around that cruel knot at your clit. I want you to soak it, I want you to drench the rope with your juice, I want you to climax for me, to give me your tightly restrained release to prove just how much you are mine, so mine. It's going to be awkward for you, and it's going to be hot.

And I'm going to be watching, right here in your mind where we meet. I'm going to be watching and thinking about how I'm going to fuck you while you're tied like that. I'm going to have you and there's nothing you can do except accept the possession when my cock pounds deep into your tight, slick pussy. I'm going to make you suck me, for hours and hours and hours. I'm going to take you up the ass so hard you're going to think you've been split in half. I'm going to take you, every way you can be taken, and you're going to take it because tied like this you don't have a choice. This isn't about whether you like it or not, honey. This is about whether I like it. I get to have you, exactly how I want you, as long as I want you, objectified, reduced to the sum of your sexual openings, desired but not considered.

And you can struggle if you want, honey. You can protest, I don't care. Because I know you, and I know deep down you love it just as much as I do, you love the surrender, you love the helpless, hapless exploitation of your body for my pleasure. And you will come for me too, but not because you like it, not even because you need it. You will come for me because it turns me on so much to watch it, and you're here for my pleasure, bound and presented. So come for me, come tied up, restrained and helpless for me. Come for me right now. *Now!*

Part Ten

    Good girl, such a good girl. You can untie yourself now, but don't think this is the end. Remember that first rope, remember karada? Next time you go out, I want you wearing it under your dress, to remind you of your place, to remind you that you're mine. And from now until forever, every time you wear that dress, I want karada under it. Because your mine, all mine.

Surf Girl

I like to dress well. I have to for work, to present the proper image, conservative and professional. I like to be attractive too, in a carefully understated way. I wear a designer blouse, good shoes, a dress skirt, and my stockings are always straight. I do attract attention, I'm pretty and I have a nice figure, but I don't flaunt it. Flaunting it is cheap, and I'm anything but cheap. I'm the same about everything. I drive a nice car but not the flashy one I could buy if I wanted to. I have a nice house in a desirable neighbourhood by the beach, but it isn't some ostentatious trophy home like some of the ones around. I have a nice boyfriend, and we have nice sex and he treats me like a princess. I like to surf on the weekends, so it's good to be by the water. My life is all sorted out.

The first place I saw the stranger was on the beach. I was going to paddle my board out to my island and surf back. It isn't really my island, but nobody goes there but me, and it has its own little beach. He was just walking down the sand, and he was looking at me, in the eye. I looked away, but when I looked back his gaze was still on mine. I turned away and went into the water and went out to my island. I don't like strangers who get too familiar. He wasn't bad looking though, and his eyes seemed kind. Eventually I caught a good wave back and made dinner and he was gone from my mind.

Or I thought he was. I recognized him the next time I saw him, two days later. He was walking down the road while I was watering my garden. I looked up and there he was, his gaze was already locked on mine. He didn't look away and I wanted him to so I just kept my eyes on his. Men can't hold my gaze for long. But he did.

"Good morning," I said, because one of us had to say something. I kept my voice polite and reserved. How dare he not look away?

"Good morning." He nodded and went past.

It was two weeks before I saw him again. Maybe he had to travel for work, maybe our paths just didn't cross. In my neighbourhood people like their privacy, we don't ask about their business. It had been a stressful two weeks. I'd had to fire my secretary, which meant dealing with the union, which I hate. I was planning on surfing the weekend away, and I was waxing my board in my front yard in my shorts and tee-shirt. It was hot and I'd brought out a jug of

Surf Girl

lemonade, just lemons and ice with a hint of sugar, very refreshing. It was the same as last time, I was concentrating on my board, and I looked up, and there he was walking along, his eyes already right there, as if he knew where mine were going to be when I looked up.

"Good morning," I said, reserved and polite again.

"Good morning." He should have kept walking, but he stopped, his eyes still locked on mine. They seemed so deep, like hypnotic pools. I wanted him to keep going but he didn't.

I couldn't just ignore him. "Would you like some lemonade?" I asked. Of course he couldn't accept, I wasn't really offering, only being polite.

"I'd like coffee," he answered. His eyes didn't waver.

Coffee? I hadn't offered him coffee. He was supposed to smile and refuse and keep walking. Didn't he know the rules? What could I do? Having offered him something to drink, it would be impolite to not get him what he wanted. I smiled. "I'll just put some on."

When I turned around our eyes broke contact, and it was like diving into a cool pool after a warm bath. I felt a fog lift that I hadn't even realized was there, my mind seemed clearer when I wasn't looking into his eyes. At the same time, I missed their inviting warmth. I went inside and he followed. I was surprised, but I couldn't say anything. I had invited him, sort of, though I hadn't intended to. It didn't scare me that he came in despite the somewhat unusual situation. His eyes were kind, it was just that his gaze was so intense.

"Do you like cream?" I asked, to keep the conversation moving.

"I do." He was looking at my kitchen table, which is a good, solid one, an antique built the way they don't build things anymore. He put his hands on it and pushed, as though testing it. "I like your table."

"Thank-you." I smiled. "I got it from..."

At that point I looked up, and his eyes were waiting for mine, right there. I was instantly back in the warm bath, and I relaxed almost at once, forgetting where I'd gotten my table from. He was so damn hypnotic!

"I'd like you to bend over, right here," he said, quite matter-of-factly, patting my table at the end near him to show me where he wanted me. I was shocked! This was too much. I didn't even know him. I was going to tell him to leave, but somehow my lips wouldn't form the words. My throat worked a moment trying to get them out, and I found myself stepping forward, moving around the table. He moved back to give me room, never taking his eyes from mine. Some part of my brain thought I could get away when I turned around to bend over. Eye contact would be broken and I could tell him to go without looking at him again, but the wall over my sink is mirrored, and when I turned around he caught my gaze with his in the mirror before I could recover myself. I bent over, exposing my ass. I couldn't believe I was doing this! It was wrong, against everything I believed in! At the same time, I found myself breathing faster, my heart pounding. He was quite good looking.

He stepped up behind me and pulled my shorts down to my knees. His hands were on my thighs, gently urging my legs apart, until my knees were trapped by my shorts. I couldn't do anything but submit to him, his eyes still held mine in the mirror. He ran a finger over my clit and up between my labia. It felt so good I couldn't repress a small moan, and perhaps I involuntarily arched my back a bit, pressed back towards him a little. I couldn't help myself, I was wet. He pressed the now slick finger against the tight ring of my anus.

"Have you ever been fucked in the ass?" he asked, in the same conversational tone he'd used to ask for coffee. I couldn't find the words to answer, and so just shook my head. *No.*

"It's going to hurt. It's supposed to."

His finger was pressing in, lubricating me with my own juices. I closed my eyes, freeing myself from his hypnotism or whatever it was, but it didn't make a difference. His finger in my ass had me paralyzed, probing me like that. It was uncomfortable and humiliating, but I couldn't summon the will to stop him. He was undoing his fly, and then I felt the swollen head of his cock pressing in right where his finger had opened me, so stiff, so hot. I was panting. He slid right into me, and it did hurt, not so much as I'd feared. I felt very full, but also very turned on.

"You're going to take it up the ass every week, to keep you in your place." His voice wasn't quite so relaxed now, it held an edge. My eyes flew open to find his gaze in the mirror. His eyes weren't kind anymore, they were steely, determined. His hands went to my hips and he began to thrust into me, taking me, claiming me as his in a way I'd never had done before. All I could do was hang on to the edge of the table. His cock swelled further, stretching me, penetrating me deeper, transforming me. If I were going to save myself from being his slave I had to do it now. I summoned all my will power to tell him to stop, but what came out of my mouth was a grunt that sounded closer to "More!" than anything else. He got harder at that, and I knew his orgasm would be huge, flooding my abused rectum with his sperm. If he came in my ass I'd be lost for sure, reshaped into his anal slut to use whenever he wanted to.

I had to stop him! I formed the word "Stop" in my mind, ran it over my lips, took a deep breath, but this time what I said was, "Harder! Please!" He did as I asked, even as my shocked brain tried to figure out how those words came out. I tried to say stop again, and this time heard myself begging. "Do it hard! Make it hurt!" That was all it took. I felt him swell further, felt his fingers digging into my hips as he came, pumping his sperm deep into my ass. His shoulders flexed, muscles tensed hard in the mirror. I could feel him throbbing so deep inside, see the pain and pleasure in my face right before my own climax hit.

Surf Girl

    I never did figure out where those words came from, but now I say them every week when he ass-fucks me. And also when I've been bad and he uses his belt.

Part Eleven

Do you know what I miss, honey? I miss hearing your voice, I miss your touch, I miss the thousand tiny intimacies a day that lovers exchange. I miss the look in your eyes when I look at you, the look that says, "I'm yours and you're mine." I miss that easy intimacy, and I miss knowing the way you feel about me.

Which is strange when you think about it, because you haven't seen me, haven't met me, and I haven't met you. And yet it isn't so strange, because we have lived in each other's fantasies for years now, we have been there always in each other's awareness, and if we haven't known each other's names that hasn't dimmed the desire, not one little bit. And now, honey, we have names. I call you honey, and let me tell you what "honey" means to me. It means sticky and sweet and natural. Honey is thick and rich and nourishing, honey is simple, straightforward and honest. Honey is rare and desirable, and like a bear who withstands a thousand stings for a taste of heaven, there's nothing I wouldn't do for my honey.

Honey – hear it, it's magical, isn't it? Honey is the perfect name for you, not your common name, not what your family or your friends call you, honey is just for me. Honey, hmmm, honey. I do miss you, honey.

And you, you know my name, from the cover of this book, but you don't use it. You call me Sir, of course you do. "Yes sir, please fuck me." "Yes sir, please whip me." "Yes sir, please hold me." "Yes sir, I miss you too." And you do miss me, when we're apart. Do you wish I were there with you, close enough to touch, to feel, to taste? You do, I know you do, because here you are, so far along in our journey together. We're so close, honey, and yet so far. And this book, seventy five thousand words squeezed from my soul, this book is my love letter written to you and cast into the world, in the certain knowledge that it will find its way into your hands.

And how do you feel about me, honey? How do you feel about the way I make you feel? I want you to tell me, I want you to write me a letter, a long letter, an intimate letter. I want to know what I do for you, I want to know how much you want me, I want to know how I've captured you like no-one else ever has. Write me, honey, and tell me those secrets you can't tell your mom or your dad or your best friend. Write me, honey, and let me know that you're out

Part Eleven

there, that you're as real as I am. Write me and show me who you are, my sweet honey, unique in all the world. I don't need eloquence and poetry, I just need you, just as you are, your words, your thoughts, your feelings, your life.

Tell me where you work and tell me how you play. Tell me where you're going, where you've been, and what you need, and what you dream. I want to know you, honey. I want to know everything there is to know about you, and only you can tell me, and the only way to do that is to write.

Don't get pen and paper yet, honey. I want you to lie back and remember first, lie back and think about what it was like the first time we were together. Were you shocked by my directness? I think you were, because where else have you read anything like this? Shocked by it, but intrigued as well, and then aroused. You do need directness, you need to know exactly where you stand, and with me you always know, which isn't to say I don't surprise you every time you turn the page. Think back to that first time you stepped through our door, set foot on our journey.

Remember the way my words washed over you, the way they swept away the rest of the world to leave you and I alone together between these sheets. Remember the rush, remember the blush, as you first realized exactly what I was doing, and then understood that there was nothing you would do, nothing you *could* do to stop it. Remember how your heart beat faster, remember how you were swept away. You couldn't wait to be alone with me, could you?

And now I'm your secret lover, always there at the back of your mind, in that secret place deep inside your mind, where everything is true. It's amazing how fast that happened, but it did. Remember it all, honey, remember it all so you can tell me about it. Show me with words what you show me with your body. Show me with words what I am to you, what I do to you. Don't edit, don't compose, don't make them fine and eloquent, just make them real, make them true, let them spill across the page. Show me your heart, show me your passion.

Show me all of you. Write now.

The Buyer

I noticed her on Monday, coming through the lobby of my office tower, dressed in expensive style, hips swinging in time to the *click-clack* of her designer shoes, her purse riding her right hip, her briefcase in her left hand. I met her gaze and held it as she passed. Does she work here? It doesn't matter. I'm on my way out as she comes in, my day too full to devote time to any woman, no matter how beautiful.

I noticed her on Wednesday, I'm coming in, she's going out, and this time I watched how she carried herself, shoulders square, head up, moving with a purposeful stride. I had a purchase to plan and by the time it was over and done I had forgotten her again.

On Friday, early morning, she reminds me, coming in when I was, and I hold the door for her.

She doesn't go through, she stops, eyes challenging. "You don't have to open the door because I'm a woman, you know."

"I didn't." I stay where I am, keep the door wide.

"No?" She raises an eyebrow. "Then why are you holding it open?"

"Because I'm a gentleman."

"Touche." She gives me half a smile and goes through, and we walk towards the waiting elevators. "You're here very early."

"I'm always here early."

"What do you do?"

"I'm a buyer." I push the button for my floor, and she pushes the button for hers.

"What do you buy?" The doors close and we start up.

I shrug. "Anything I can sell for a profit."

"Such as?"

"Companies, mostly."

"Leveraged buyouts?"

I nod. "Usually."

She smiles at that, reaches into her purse, takes out her wallet, gives me her card. "Let me know if you need some help."

The Buyer

I read it. I've heard her name before, and her credentials are impressive. "Perhaps I can use you." I take out my own wallet, give her my card. "Come by my office and we'll see."

"What time?"

"Seven, tonight."

"Do you always work late, too?"

"Always."

She nods, smiles, as the elevator stops and the doors open for her floor. "Well, I'll see you then."

I go through my day, calls and meetings, opportunities gained and lost, and at seven PM the night girl calls from the front desk.

"Your seven o'clock is here to see you."

I look up. It takes me a moment to remember the name on her card, though her face is unforgettable. "Send her in."

I get up as she comes through the door, shake her hand, usher her into the plush leather chair across from my desk.

"Thank-you for coming in so late."

"We do whatever we have to do for our clients. That's what makes us the best." She opens her briefcase. "I spent some time researching your operation this afternoon. I think there are four key areas where we can…"

I hold a hand to stop her in mid-sentence. "I'd like to buy your jacket."

"My jacket?" Her face registers surprise. "Why?"

"Does the reason matter?"

"I can't sell it, it's matched to the skirt."

"Of course you can sell it. Name a price high enough to cover a new skirt as well."

"Seriously?"

"I never joke about deals."

"Fair enough." She names a price. It's high, but then her suit is custom tailored, and she deserves a profit. I open a drawer, count out hundred dollar bills. She takes them, takes off her jacket and hands it over. I write out a receipt. *One grey designer jacket, used, purchased at 7:10PM.* I add the date, fill in the amount. "Sign here please."

She laughs and takes my pen, "I doubt you'll get a tax deduction."

"Probably not."

"I hope the rest of our deal is this easy."

"I do too." I smile and put the jacket in the bottom drawer of my desk. "I'd like your blouse too, please."

"What?" She looks at me in shock.

"I'd like you to give me your blouse."

Her face is suddenly hard. "I sold the jacket, not the blouse."

"So name another price."

She stands up. "I think I should leave."

"If you think so."

"Do you have any idea how rude that is?" Her briefcase closes with a sharp *snap*. "I thought you were a gentleman."

"All's fair in love and business. How much do you want for it?"

She snorts derisively. "It's not for sale."

"Everything is for sale, the only question is price." I start counting out hundred dollar bills. "I'm thinking of a number. If your blouse is on my desk before I reach it, we have a deal." I start counting the money out, slowly, steadily.

She looks at me, cold and hostile. "I'm not a prostitute."

"I'm buying your blouse, not you." I keep adding bills to the pile, one by one.

"Who do you think you are?" Her voice is still angry, but she hasn't left yet.

"It doesn't matter who I am. It doesn't matter who you are. All that matters is whether we can make a deal."

"You've got a lot of nerve."

"I have to, to do what I do."

She nods slowly, considering at the growing pile of money. I'm adding to it more slowly now. "Just the blouse?"

"Just the blouse."

She looks at the pile. I add a hundred and wait. After a long pause I add another. It's already twice what I paid for her jacket. A longer pause, and then another.

"Okay," she says at last, and starts undoing buttons. I stop counting and watch while she shrugs it off. Her breasts are high and firm, well rounded beneath her white lace bra, and her large nipples poke through the sheer fabric in tempting outline. She tosses the blouse on my desk. "I hope that's worth it." Her tone is half mocking.

"It is." I take the blouse, dump it into the bottom drawer of my desk, then push the stack of bills over to her, appreciating the view. "Very nice."

She sits down again, takes the cash, riffles through it, and puts it in her briefcase. "I think that was the easiest money I ever made." She leans back, perfectly comfortable half undressed. She's knows the power of her figure, and she's enjoying this tangible validation of it.

"Deals only work if they're profitable for both sides." I make out another receipt, and she signs it.

"I agree, now to get back to the key points I've..." She trails off as I start counting out another pile of money. "What's that for?"

"Your skirt."

She looks at me. "You're quite the piece of work, aren't you?"

The Buyer

I meet her gaze, still counting. "I know what I want, I know how to get it."

"You should know, I'm not wearing underwear."

"No?" I raise an eyebrow.

"Just garters." She gives me a sly half-smile. "I think that should raise the price, don't you?"

"It's a single-bid auction," I answer. "You'll never know if I've changed my offer."

"I have confidence that you will."

I don't answer, I just keep adding bills to the pile, each one coming more slowly than the last. Her hands go unconsciously to the button at the waist of her skirt, her fingers playing with it, nervously. When I see that, I know she's mine, it's just a matter of time now. She nibbles her lip, nervous. She's wondering how high I'll go. She makes a lot of money, but there's a lot of money on the table, enough that she wants it, and she doesn't want me to stop before she takes it.

I keep my gaze on her face. Greed and fear, those twin demon-gods of the market, fight for the upper hand in her eyes. She wavers, licks her lips, looking at the money, at me, at the money again. To her credit she holds out for a very large sum indeed, but finally the button comes free, the short zipper slides down. As advertised, she isn't wearing any underwear. The straps of her garter belt form an attractive frame for the triangular thatch of her pubic hair, and her expensive stockings earn their price in the way they show off her long, smooth thighs. She picks up the skirt from the floor, puts it on the desk. I drop it in my drawer with her blouse and jacket, and slide the stack of hundreds over to her. She takes it and puts it in her briefcase with the rest, then sits back down in the chair, crosses her legs, and manages somehow to maintain the same professional poise that she had fully clothed.

I present her with a third receipt for her signature. "Now what?" she asks, challenging.

"Now I want you to stand up, bend over, and put your nose right here." I tap the edge of my desk in front of her.

She shakes her head. "No. I'm not going that far. I'm not a prostitute."

"Then I won't insult you by offering money."

She smiles a cool smile. "It's been an interesting game, but we're finished now. Is there anything else I can do for you? In a professional capacity?"

"No, just stand up and put your nose where I told you to. I want to see your cunt."

Her smile vanishes. "I think I will be going after all."

"As you wish."

She stands up, puts out a hand. "I'd like my clothes back, please."

I laugh a small laugh. "They're mine now."

"I don't think you understand." Her eyes are suddenly angry. "This game is over, and I want my clothes back."

I shake my head. "You sold them to me, at a very generous price. I'm keeping them."

Her lips compress into a thin line, and she comes around the desk. There's a brief moment when she realizes she'll have to bend down to open my bottom drawer. She compromises by squatting, and I watch as she pulls at it to find it locked.

"Open it." Her voice is tight. "Now."

I shake my head again. "No."

"You want your money back?" She goes back around the desk, grabs her briefcase, snaps it open, tosses the stacked bills on my desk. "There's your money."

"No."

She looks at me, her hard, angry eyes boring into mine. "You want a profit, is that it? You tell me how much, I'll write a cheque."

I shake my head again. "What I want is for you to bend over, right here, so I can see your cunt." I smile. "Or rather, more of your cunt."

She sees where I'm looking, and reflexively moves a hand in front of her crotch. "This isn't funny."

"No, it's business."

"I'll scream rape."

"Suit yourself." I hold up the receipts. "Here's my proof that it isn't. I'll sue you bankrupt for false accusation."

"You won't win."

"You won't either, and the case will be very public. How much is your reputation worth?"

She looks at me, long and hard. "You son of a bitch. You god-damned son of a bitch."

I shrug. "I didn't get where I am by playing nice in the sandbox." I point to my phone. "Feel free to call someone."

She doesn't drop her gaze. "You know damn well I'm not going to do that."

I nod. "I do. I just want it to be very clear in your own mind that you have a choice. You had a choice when I offered to buy your jacket and another choice with your blouse, and another with your skirt, and you have a choice right now."

"Some choice," she snorts.

"You know how leveraged buyouts work. It isn't that they want to give up the company, it's that you've bought enough of it to take control."

"Is that what you think you've done?"

177

The Buyer

"I suppose we're going to find out." I lean forward, gather the scattered hundred dollar bills into a single stack and put it at the edge of the desk. "Now I'd like you to put your nose right here." I tap the pile of money.

"And if I don't?"

"Then I'm going to close the office and go home."

"You'd really let me walk out of here naked? What about your receptionist? And the doorman? What will they think?"

"I don't care what they think."

She looks at me. "You really don't, do you?"

I lean back. "Let's make a deal. You do everything I want for the next hour. If you do, when it's over, I'll make sure you leave here decently covered, and nobody will ever, ever know what happened here."

"You're a real free-wheeling bastard, do you know that?"

"Do we have a deal?"

She looks at me with venom in her eyes, then slowly stands up, bends over and puts her nose down on the stack of bills.

"I'll take that as a yes." Her face is blushing furious red with her humiliation and she still refuses to answer. I get up, come around the desk, make myself comfortable in the plush leather chair she's just vacated, admiring her curves. She obviously works out, her waist is tight, her thighs toned. Her garter straps bisect her ass cheeks, providing the perfect frame for her pussy as she offers it to me so beautifully. I'm instantly drunk with the sight of her, intoxicated, overcome with physical need. I want to fuck her on the spot, but I've paid high for my prize and I'm going to take my time enjoying it. There's the slightest hint of moisture on the lips of her pussy. Despite her anger and her resistance, it's arousing for her to have her control taken away like this. I don't say anything, so her imagination can run wild.

She's drawn to intensity, drawn to the edge, everyone in her profession is. That's why she wasn't able to leave when I made my opening offer. It wasn't that she wasn't insulted, it was that she couldn't refuse the challenge it implied. I reach a hand up, point a finger at the center of her cunt, move it forward. She gasps as I touch her, her body jerking, her hips coming back reflexively, sinking my finger into her warm, sticky-slick depths. I slide my finger steadily in, and she stifles a moan as she accepts it.

"Do you have to do that?" She sounds aggrieved, but her wetness is proof that she isn't.

"No." I chuckle. "I just want to."

I slide my finger out, heavily coated with the evidence of her arousal, move it up a fraction of an inch and slide it into her tight, rosy anus. I do it hard and fast, not giving her time to relax. She gives a little mew of discomfort. She doesn't like this, which is exactly why I'm doing it. I want her to feel degraded because I want her to know that I own her. I want her to *feel* that I own her. She learns the lesson immediately and physically, unable to prevent her back from arching, instinctively giving me better access as I violate her ass.

"You aren't allowed to orgasm," I tell her.

"As if I would," her words are defiant, but there's an undercurrent of arousal to them. I have her just where I want her.

"You'll be punished if you do."

"I'm being punished now." She doesn't quite manage to sound annoyed.

As she says it I pull my finger out of her and push two back in, wringing an anguished cry from her throat, and a second later she's coming, hard, her body betraying her resolve in that single instant. Her hips come back, fucking her ass onto my fingers as her no-longer-virgin anal ring squeezes them with muscular rhythm. My cock swells larger still, I'm going to enjoy this. I'm going to enjoy it a lot.

Her orgasm goes on and on as she screams and writhes on my impaling digits, and her pubic hair is soaked with the juices squeezed from her clenching cunt. When she starts to slow down I push a third finger into her, stretching her wider, reminding her of what she's here for, what she is. Her second orgasm hits her with even more force than the first, and I pump her ass hard while she begs for more. Her resistance, has completely dissolved. She is so mine, so very mine.

I force her through a third orgasm, and then a fourth, and after that they blur together, following each other so closely there's no point in counting. Before I'm done she's begging me to stop, but I don't stop, not until her muscles are sore from repeated contraction, until her voice is hoarse, until her body just won't go on. Finally she just lies there, skin flushed, hair tangled, exhausted and gasping for air. The neat stack of bills has been scattered all over the floor, and she's totally spent, but we're not done yet. We've only just begun.

"You're a bad girl," I tell her. She doesn't respond.

"You're a bad girl," I repeat, and grab a luxuriant handful of hair. I pull her head up, forcing her back to arch. "Aren't you?" She still doesn't answer and I pull harder. "*Aren't you?*"

"Y...yes..." she stammers, her voice quaking. Her resistance is gone now, shattered.

"Yes what?"

"Yes, I'm a bad girl," she manages to whisper.

I bring my hand down on her ass, hard, and the slap of flesh on flesh is gunshot loud. "Yes, what?"

"Yes, sir," she yelps. "Yes, sir, I'm a bad girl." I smile. She's a quick study.

"Why are you a bad girl?"

"I... I... I came when I wasn't allowed to."

I yank on her hair and she gasps, her eyes wide. "Sir. I came when I wasn't allowed to. Sir."

The Buyer

I relax my grip a little. She understands her place now. "Why else?"

"And because I sold my clothing for money. Sir."

"And what does that make you?"

"Oh God..."

I tighten my grip again, refusing to let her avoid the question.

"Oh God, please don't make me say it... "

With my free hand I unbuckle my belt. Her eyes widen as the clasp jangles, widen further as it slithers out of the loops, twisting like a live snake in my hand. I double it, with the buckle and the free end together in my hand, and raise it over her vulnerable bottom cheeks. "Why are you a bad girl? Why did you sell your clothes?"

"Please no... please no..."

I bring the belt down with enough force to make it whistle, cracking it over her cheeks. "Why?"

"Please no..." Her words are tight around the pain in her voice.

I strap her again, right across the rounded crease where her thighs join her buttocks. There's already an angry red welt rising where my first strike hit home. "Why?" I repeat the question.

"No... no..." She thrashes her head back and forth, pulling her hair against my grip, but she's too exhausted to really fight.

"Why?" I bring the belt down. "Why?" I bring it down again. "Why?" The punctuating smacks echo against the walls.

"Because..." The word is torn from her throat, and she presses her lips together to hold back the words that follow it, squeezes her eyes shut to contain the building tears.

"Why?" I put muscle into the strokes. "Why?"

"Because... because I'm a cocktease." The dam breaks and the words come out in a torrent. "Because I wanted to tease you and make you frustrated."

I swing the belt harder as she speaks, encouraging her to full confession, scourging purification from her struggling flesh. "And why did you want that?"

"Because I'm a stuck-up bitch who teases everyone and gets away with it."

I put down the belt but keep a firm grip on her hair. I let my free hand rest on her swollen, reddened ass, enjoying the heat radiating from it, and her small flinches as I caress the tender flesh. "So what should I do with such a bad girl?"

"Punish me." A sharp yank on her hair reminds her. "Sir. Punish me, sir."

"And how should I punish you?"

"Anything, sir. Whip my pussy, whip my tits, make me crawl, make me do what you want, make me beg for it. Only please make it hurt, I need it to hurt, hard and deep."

"Tell me more," I say, reaching under her to squeeze a nipple, hard, harder, harder still. "Tell me that you need it."

"Oh, I need it." She moans at the pain. "I need it, sir, I need to be put in my place, I need to be taken, I need to be used. Make me take it, make me take it till I can't take it anymore, and then make me take it deeper, harder. Punish me, mark me, and then come on my face, up my ass, anywhere, anything. Make me respect your cock, make me worship it, I'll be good for you, sir, I promise I will."

"Convince me."

She spreads her legs wider, splitting her swollen, soaking vulva, then reaches around behind her, spreads her cheeks to offer me everything. "Right here, it's all yours, bought and paid for. I'm your slut, I'm your whore. Fuck me, please fuck me,"

I crack the belt up between her legs, aiming for her ripe and rigid clit. She yelps but holds her position. "What do you say?"

She knows the answer, she knows it not just by heart but from her heart, from her secret dreams, now as exposed as her ass. "Thank you sir, please whip me harder, I'm your dirty little slut."

I smile. There's always hidden wealth in any deal, but I never dreamed I'd find such treasure here. I punish her clit again.

"Thank you sir, please whip me harder, I'm your dirty little slut." Her words are drenched in pain but her cunt is drenched in juice and her clit is standing hard, begging for more. Yes she needs it, she needs everything she's begging for, she's needed it for years. She needs it almost as badly as I need to give it to her, so I give it to her full force, full strength, aiming for her offered anus, and I earn another yelp.

"Thank you sir, please whip me harder, I'm your dirty little slut." Again. "Thank you sir, please whip me harder, I'm your dirty little slut." She's crying now, but she isn't moving, taking all I have to give. "Thank you sir, please whip me harder, I'm your dirty little slut."

I pick up the pace, not letting her finish, blurring her words with pain and need. "Thank you sir, thank you sir, thank you sir, please. Please whip me harder, whip me harder, whip me harder. Please whip me harder, I'm your dirty little slut, little slut, little slut, slut, slut, slut." It turns into her mantra as I etch my name onto her ass with the lash of my belt.

Red lines blossom on her smooth, creamy skin, and every single one sends a surge to my cock. It's hurting now itself, raging for release, pounding with my pulse, with its need. It's desperate now, lunging at my straining zipper, hungry to impose its will on the open cunt in front of it, perhaps even another man's cunt. What are the odds such a woman is single? Not high, but here she is in front of me, pussy presented with adulterous eagerness for whatever I desire. My heartbeat is a drumbeat in my ears, in my mind and I can't see straight, can't think straight, my brain contains one single thought, to consummate her conquest.

The Buyer

She is moaning, crying, bucking, writhing, stripped to her essentials, supplicating to my cock. I'm going to fuck her, she knows I am, stallion style, slamming it in, impaling her with no regard for her pain or her pleasure. I'm going to fuck her, despoil her, degrade her and she's going to take it, take every last inch of it, she's going to take it again and again. I'm going to fuck her, and in fucking her I'm going to own her, violate her, humiliate her, take possession of her very soul and she knows that too.

She knows it, she needs it, and she's getting it, hard and good. And she's beyond crying now, completely, gone beyond words, beyond thought, beyond any awareness but the submission I've inflicted on her surrendered pussy. Her tears have been her penance, full payment for her sins, extracted stroke by stroke from her ass. Her tears are real, as is her pain, but she's had worse punishment than what I'm giving her. She's lived for years the formless hell of asking, begging, pleading for what she needs, of offering all she has, all she is and getting – not a thing. She's done her time, untamed and unrestrained, a wild thing lost and hungry, but she's feeding now, feasting. She needs to be objectified, and I can't fucking stand it anymore. I drop the belt, rip out my cock, grab her hips and split her slit with it, hot and slick and tight, tight, tight. The teeth of my zipper shreds her skin, tearing at it where it's red, hurting her as I hurt her, as I slam her tender cervix to make her know she's mine.

She screams as I force her wider, pumping her full of flesh, hands around her waist, in total control. She's my fucking dirty little slut and I fucking love it, watching her punished pussy take it fully deep. I fuck her fast and fuck her slow, making her feel it, making her beg for more through her tears. "Fuck me, fuck me, fuck your slut, use me like a whore, like your whore, like your hole, please, sir, use me, make me fucking take it, make it hurt, make me yours."

And I do it, do it to her, because I need it, need it bad. And I fuck her for forever, fucking fill her, flood her cunt. My hot sperm overwhelms her and she screams out her own pleasure, cunt contracting hard, hard, hard. And the lights go dim and wavy and my hips will not stop thrusting, my body won't stop fucking until the lights turn red. I nearly pass out from the pleasure, and when I recover myself my balls are sore, literally wrung dry in a single ejaculation, the evidence of my excess spilling down her thighs.

"Thank-you, sir." Her voice is soft, relaxed. I stay inside her, enjoying her. I have all the time in the world to do that now. Whatever she was before, she's mine now. Bought and paid for.

Part Twelve

Today's lesson is about obedience. You've always been good at getting your way, haven't you, honey? When you can't beat the system with brains you beat it with big eyes and a little flirtation. What you haven't been good at is doing what you're told, and why should you be? Nobody's ever really made you, have they?

Well that's about to change.

So the first thing you're going to learn is how to undress. This isn't about a strip tease, honey, this is about getting your clothes off in a smooth and simple way. What, did you expect to be wearing those clothes for long? Not this time, honey. In a moment I'm going to tell you "Strip," and when I do you're going to start at the top, and work your way down, blouse and bra, put them neatly aside. No folding, no hanging up, but no tossing on the floor either. Just get them out of the way where they won't get wrinkled. Are you wearing a skirt or pants? It doesn't matter, that's coming off next, and then panties. Shoes off, stockings off, and you're naked. I want it quick and smooth. Turn the page when you're done.

Clear on that?

Strip.

Part Twelve

And now that I have you naked, the next thing you're going to learn is how to stand, because you don't know how. You don't stand straight enough, honey. You don't do justice to your lovely figure. Just put your feet shoulder width apart, clasp your hands together in the small of your back, square your shoulders, pull your stomach in and raise your chin to keep your head level. See how that shows off your tits, see how that emphasizes your waist. Pick a spot on the wall and just stare at it, and hold that position five minutes. That's one hundred heartbeats. It's restful, in its fashion, to stand like that with nothing to do but stare at the wall and count. It's a decision free environment, relaxing after a long day, so we're going to call this position "Rest". When I tell you "Rest," you just move to this position, and then you'll wait one hundred heartbeats, and then you'll turn the page.

Ready?

Rest.

Part Twelve

Good girl, and that was nicer than you might have expected, and longer too. Take a deep breath and think about how nice that was, then we're going to learn the next position, which is "Attention," just like in the army. When I tell you, "Attention," all you're going to do is move your left foot in until your heels touch, and move your hands down to your sides. Curl your fingers tight, with thumb pressed down on your index finger, and then align your thumbs along your thighs, right where the seam of your pants would be, if you had pants.

Of course you don't have pants, honey. You're naked for me, and you're going to be standing in this position to be inspected, and corrected on your posture, on your demeanour, on your attitude. I'm there with you, I'm watching you, in just that special way, and you're going to be on display. Your tits are going to be well presented like this, and your tingling nipples, and I can see how they're crinkling erect. Your ass is going to be presented, available to be squeezed or smacked or spread. Even your cunt will be presented, though not as presented as it will be later, and your swelling clit will be oh-so visible, oh, so available. Yeah this turns you on, honey, this makes your breathing come quicker, your heart beat faster. This gets to you, and you can't wait to be put in this position and put in your place at the same time.

Think about what goes into the position of "Attention." Get it clear in your mind so when you do it, you do it right. You're going to stay in it for one hundred heartbeats. One hundred heartbeats focused on that spot on the wall. One hundred heartbeats, honey, and then turn the page.

Attention.

Part Twelve

And how does that feel, my obedient little girl. It's calming, relaxing, to have no decisions to make. Calming, relaxing, to be focused like that. It's calming, relaxing, and at the same time arousing, because you know your decisions are mine now, because you know, deep inside your mind, that deep inside, you're mine.

Deep breath in, clear your thoughts, and ready for the next instruction. You're going to do it one hundred heartbeats

Rest.

Part Twelve

And now we're going to move you back. When you hear "Attention," you move your hands back down to your thighs, fingers curled, thumbs back where the seam of your pants would be, back straight, stomach in, tits out. Understand how these positions go together. From Rest you can move to Attention, from Attention you can move to Rest. Each one is a different way to display your body, every one offers a different level of control over your being. Each makes you mine in just one more degree. Be ready to count, one hundred heartbeats. Be ready to give yourself to me.
Attention.

Part Twelve

Hands in the small of your back, legs shoulder width apart, chin up, stomach in, tits out. One hundred heartbeats and turn the page.
Rest.

Part Twelve

Heels together, arms straight down by your sides, fingers curled, thumbs running vertically down your thighs. Keep your chin up, eyes focused on that single spot on the wall. One hundred heartbeats and turn the page.
Attention.

Part Twelve

Very good, honey. Now that you're getting good at this part, it's time to learn a new position, and the position is "Kneel." There are rules to this. You're told to Kneel only from the position of Attention, and when you are told, you're going to drop to your knees, right knee going down first, left leg going down last, and otherwise it's exactly the same as Attention. Back straight, stomach in, tits out. Sound familiar, honey? Head level, eyes locked on the wall. Obedience is what I want from you right now. Obedience is what I'm going to get. One hundred heartbeats.

Kneel.

Part Twelve

Now to go back to Attention from Kneel is very simple. Right leg up first, then left leg, and it's still back straight, stomach in, chin up, head level, eyes locked on that spot on the wall. One hundred heartbeats.
Attention.

Part Twelve

One hundred heartbeats.
Kneel.

Part Twelve

Very good honey, very obedient.
Attention.

Part Twelve

Kneel.

Part Twelve

Attention.

Part Twelve

Kneel.

Part Twelve

And now it's going to get good. The next position is called "Present." And all that's going to happen when you hear "Present" is you're going to bend at the waist, bring your body forward, with your forearms forward and your right cheek on the ground. Think about how it's going to feel to be commanded into that position, honey. Think how it's going to feel with your ass in the air and your pussy presented. Think about how exposed you're going to be. Think about how you could be explored, examined, probed, fucked. Think about how you could be whipped, on your ass, on your cunt, on your rigid little clit, on your tempting little anal ring.

Think about how much you're mine. One hundred heartbeats.

Present.

Part Twelve

One hundred heartbeats.
Kneel.

Part Twelve

One hundred heartbeats.
Present.

Part Twelve

And there's one more command, honey. One more word to complete your obedience training, complete your conversion from independent woman to sexual slave. And that command is "Open." When I tell you "Open," all you're going to do is move your right leg eighteen inches to the right, nothing more, nothing less. And you're going to be so open for me then, your wet and swollen slit parted and glistening. You'll be on display in the most fundamental way, and the scent of sex is going to waft from your cunt to fill the room. You're going to be mine so completely, honey. You're going to be compelled to it, driven to it, you aren't going to be able to help yourself. And in fact all you wish right now is that I would stop talking and get on with it, allow you to spread yourself, present yourself, to prove to me just how much you're mine.

So do it, honey. One hundred heartbeats.

Open.

Part Twelve

And you're so hot like this, honey. You're such an easy, eager slut for me, the total sex slave, put through your paces, obedient and obeying, pliant and compliant. You're ready for me now, ready for me to put my cock in you, ready for me to fuck you, in your cunt, in your mouth, in your ass. You're ready for me to tie you, to whip you, to spurt my sperm all over you. You're ready to be used and abused, anything so long as you're not ignored, anything, so long as the deep need burning in your womb is satisfied, anything, as long as you know that you're pleasing my cock.

Anything.

And so I want just one thing from you, honey, and that is your orgasm in this position, I want the physical proof of your desire. I want you to slide a hand down to your clit in the certain knowledge that moving out of position is going to earn you a slice of the riding crop across your tight stretched ass. I want you to do that because you need the release too much to care about the pain, and I want your fingers going up and down on the rigid, bursting nub of your clit so fast they'd be just a blur on any porn director's camera.

I want you to give it all up for me, honey, in this most submissive of submissive positions, and I want you to be saying my name when you do come, screaming it out, begging for it, begging for it harder. Just think about how you look to me right now, honey, face down, ass up, wet and spread and pleading for it, obedient to whatever I say. Just think about how hard my cock is right now, honey. Think about how much you're mine, and think about how good it's going to be when your climax hits.

And it's going to hit. Right now.

Now!

Part Twelve

Good girl, such a good girl. You can relax now, we're done. But I want you to go over this exercise until you know your positions by heart. I want you to go over them every night, before you go to bed. *Strip, rest, attention, kneel, present, open.* Every night, honey, because you're mine. And at the end, when you're naked, kneeling, presented, open, I want your climax, offered up like your pussy is now, a ritual supplication of your body and your mind. I want that, honey, because I want you to be ready for me, whenever I want you, however I want you. I want that because there's nothing I want more than you. Right now, and always.

The Writer

The train wheels pound steadily in the darkness and cold rain streaks the windows, blurring city lights into a semi-surrealistic landscape. The car is almost deserted. Across from me an expensively dressed businessman pores over no-doubt important files. A few seats down a young woman in a dress skirt and a jacket that was probably warm enough this morning is immersed in a book. My reflection stares back at me, half mirrored over the cityscape, showing a man I somehow have trouble recognizing. My journey is almost at an end, three planes, two trains, and a continent ago. I have two more station stops and a cab ride left. I've been traveling sixteen hours, grabbing sleep where I can, eating overpriced and under-nourishing food, occupying my time with books, with shallow conversation with people I'll never see again, with the idle contemplation of the world seen from far, far above.

I had intended to put some work into my book, but my laptop remains in my carry-on bag, untouched since takeoff. In sixteen hours of enforced idleness I can produce ten thousand words of undying prose, given only inspiration. Inspiration was lacking for the trans-ocean flight, for the entire journey, has been lacking for a year now. My production file remains as empty as the house I'm returning to. The reason is simple. Emily is gone, gone so completely it sometimes seems she was never there at all.

It has never been easy, this past year, but it's not quite so hard when I'm away. Because of that I've made a point of being away, I tell my publisher I'm promoting my previous book, but in reality I'm avoiding the one I should be writing now. This last trip has been six months living out of a suitcase, forty cities, twenty-four thousand frequent flyer miles. I've signed autographs and given lectures, gone to launch parties and reading circles. I've shaken hands, been interviewed on every form of media the modern world allows. The only thing I haven't done is forgotten, and the only problem is *away* never lasts, and the hardest thing of all is coming home to an empty house.

Everyone loved my last book, everyone wants to know when the next one is coming out. "Soon," I tell them, which I know is a lie. I'm supposed to be done by now, and my agent calls me weekly for updates. My publisher has given up calling.

The Writer

The train slows, glides into the next station, they announce the stop. The businessman closes up his briefcase and gets off. Outside snow is starting to blend into the rain, heavy wet flakes sticking to the window to melt there, to slide down and away and off the bottom edge of the window to vanish into the darkness. I consider pulling out the laptop and at least going through the motions of writing, but there's no point. The empty screen, the beckoning keyboard, these are an exquisite form of self-torture that I'm simply too tired to indulge in right now.

The doors close and the train slowly accelerates, the wheels beating against the rails in a rising rhythm. I watch as we start to outrace cars on the highway that parallels the tracks and I think about their drivers, each isolated in their own metal and glass cocoon, each immersed in their private thoughts as they drive. All of us are sharing this slice of the night in total anonymity, all of us are united only in our desire to be elsewhere, quickly.

My problem is, I never get to elsewhere, and that desire never goes away. I've been running from myself, running from my memories, and I'm running out of places to run. An industrial park slides past, tanks and hoppers and pipes at a chemical plant, thousands of concrete highway barriers ranked with military precision at a huge industrial building where, I presume, they make highway barriers. I'm somehow surprised that there's a market for them large enough to support a plant this big, but the evidence is in front of me. It's a thought I've had before, I've taken this train on this same route dozens, maybe hundreds of times. I recognize the landmarks, I know that the level crossing comes after the lumberyard, and then we're into a mile or so of semi-suburbia before the bridge over the ravine where the park is, and yet if you asked me to describe any of it when I wasn't looking at it, I'd be able to give only the vaguest description. The mind is a funny thing.

If you asked me to describe Emily it would be different. Every detail of her is burned into my heart. I can close my eyes and feel the texture of her hair, and see the cluster of freckles on her lower back. I know about the tiny, odd bump on the back of her right ear. I can hear her voice, see her smile, taste her kiss. Could she only have been my imagination, so real and so detailed? There have been other women since Emily. None of them have been as real as her. None have done anything more than highlight the place in my life she no longer fills. It isn't her fault that she's gone, it isn't their fault they aren't her. Could I really have dreamed her, when my imagination can't conjure a single word?

The night slides by with a million strangers out there in it. Surely, somewhere in that teeming multitude, there must be another woman as brilliant, as beautiful, as alive as she was. I sometimes wonder if it's even possible to love, truly love, more than once in your life. You can dream of love, but can you love a dream? The mind is a funny thing.

The wheels pound, the miles pass, and then we're rolling into another station, the last stop, my stop, end of the line. I collect my baggage and get up when the doors open. As I stand up I notice the woman looking at me. She's attractive, mid-to-upper twenties, well dressed in conservative style. I give her a polite smile and go out onto the platform, leaning against the wind as the sleet whips into my face. I hurry into the warmth of the station, get out my phone and call a cab as I walk.

"Excuse me?"

I look around. It's her.

"Yes?"

"Can I ask your name?"

I tell her.

She smiles. "I thought I recognized you." She holds out the book she was reading and a pen. "Can I get you to sign this?"

I take the book. It isn't the one she was reading, and it isn't the one I've been signing for the last six months, it's another one, with another name on the black and red cover. I look at her. "This isn't me."

"No, but it's your pseudonym."

My eyebrows go up. "Not a lot of people know that."

"It's an open secret."

"Only if you care to do the research."

She nods. "I saw your talk at the university, last year."

"Who should I sign it to?"

She tells me.

"Is there anything in particular you'd like me to write?"

"Anything you want." She smiles.

I think of something clever, sign the book and hand it back. "Did you like it?"

She hesitates. "It was… intense..."

Intense. Yes, it was intense. There's a reason I used a pseudonym, used a different agent and a different publisher. This is the only thing I've managed to write since Emily, and unlike what I'm supposed to be writing, the words in this book came spilling out of me like blood from a mortal wound. It doesn't fit in with anything else I've written. It doesn't fit in with anything anyone else has written. I don't want friends and family knowing that I wrote it. Some things are so personal you can only share them with strangers.

"But did you like it?" I ask.

She blushes, looks down, her voice dropping a few decibels. "Yes. Yes, I liked it very much."

"I'm glad." I allow myself a smile at her embarrassment. I know as much about her as she knows about me now, perhaps too much for strangers to know about each other when they're standing face to face. A cab pulls up in front of the station. "This is me," I say. "It was nice meeting you."

"Listen, are you... I mean... Where are you going? Maybe we can share...?"

"I'm going to dinner," I say it as I decide it. I don't want to go back to my empty house, not yet. "Anywhere downtown works for me."

"I live downtown."

The driver opens the trunk and we throw our bags in. I hold the door open for her as she gets into the warm darkness of the back of the cab. I give the driver my destination and she gives him hers, and we talk about the miserable weather, and then the political situation, and a few other trivialities. We're well enough acquainted by the time the cab pulls up in front of my restaurant that it seems natural for me to invite her in with me, and natural for her to accept.

We go in, are seated, and continue talking about everything, about nothing. She is, perhaps, just one more passing travel acquaintance, a person who'll fill a few hours of my life and then vanish without trace. Still, she is pleasant and intelligent company, witty and articulate, and there is, unspoken between us, the inherent possibility that there might be more to come. Dinner is ordered, arrived, is eaten, dessert follows, and then coffee, and then she asks me a question.

"So is your book based on real life?" She almost manages to be casual in asking.

I smile. "Real life is all I have to base it on."

"I mean, have you done... any of those things?"

I nod. "At some time or other." I watch her face, watch her eyes as she tries to ask the next question. I save her the struggle by turning her first question around. "Have you?"

"No."

"Would you like to?"

She looks at me, our gazes lock. She bites her lower lip and it seems to take forever before she answers. I give her points for what I see in her face while I wait. There is excitement, but also cool calculation. She wants what I can give her, but she's also not going to rush into something based purely on desire. She's a smart girl, and that just makes her more attractive. Eventually she nods. "Yes."

I beckon the waiter, give him my credit card and get him to call a cab for us.

"Are we going to your place?" she asks at the door while we wait for another cab.

"Yours is closer."

"But don't you need..."

"Everything I need is already in your mind."

Her eyebrows go up at that, but she doesn't say anything. The cab ride is short, it would have been a pleasant walk in better weather. I put my hand on her knee and open her legs, slide my hand up her thigh, under her skirt to find her panties soaking wet. I smile to myself. It's going to be a good night. I make idle conversation with the cab driver while I explore her cunt and she squirms on the seat, biting her lip to avoid gasping and moaning. We pull up in front of her building and I tell the driver to wait.

"Are you going to be that fast?" she asks, half teasing, half questioning.

"We'll see."

She's practically skipping with excitement as she leads me in, leads me up a flight of stairs to a small but well appointed two bedroom apartment. I kiss her at the threshold gently, briefly, not nearly enough, and then let her show me her space. It's nice, hardwood floors, slightly messier than I would have expected, breakfast dishes still in the sink, books piled on the coffee table and on bookshelves against one wall, an expensive stereo system and racks and racks of compact discs. She's a book lover and a music lover, and I take a moment to glance at the titles in her collection.

The second room is her study, and her desk is there with her computer, and as she's showing me I take her hands and guide them down so her palms are flat on her desk. She stops talking, and her eyes are big and wide. I undo my belt. It sounds like a snake as I slide it out through the loops. She gasps, looking back over her shoulder to see what I'm doing.

"It works like this," I say, pulling up her skirt. "You're going to get twelve with the belt. You keep your hands on the desk. If you take them off, we're done."

"Done?"

"Done. I'll go home, the cab is waiting. No fault, no blame, no hard feelings."

She nods. "Okay." There's a tremble in her voice.

"You're going to count them."

She nods again. "Yes."

"Yes, sir," I remind her, because she expects to be reminded.

"Yes, sir."

Her underwear is basic black, no obstacle to the belt. I raise it and pause to admire the curve of her luscious buttocks, her trim waist. There have been other women since Emily, but there hasn't been this. I haven't had the emotional strength. Do I have it now?

I bring the belt down to snap across her ass. She yelps, gasps and almost brings her hands off the desk in sheer reflex. At the last moment she manages to keep her fingertips down.

"One. Sir."

The Writer

I slash the belt down again. "Two, sir." The pain is clear in her voice, but her hands stay flat this time.

I swing it again, harder. "Three, sir." She's anguished, and angry red lines are swelling on the curve of her ass.

Again. "Four, sir." It becomes clear that I'll be sending the cab away empty.

"Five, sir." With a sort of detached surprise I can feel my erection swelling hard against my zipper.

"Six, sir... Please..."

I bring the belt down again before she has time to ask me to stop.

"Please..."

I smack her again, full force this time, and suddenly she's crying, but her hands stay flat on her desk.

"Please..."

"Keep counting," I tell her, and bring the belt across the crease where her buttocks join her thighs.

"Ni...Nine, sir."

"You left off at six."

"Oh jeeze, *please*..." I interrupt her plea with another smack of the belt. She screams and sobs and her hands still stay flat. "Seven, sir."

I strike again, letting the tip of the belt find the cleft of her cunt. She jumps. "Eight, sir."

Again, "Nine, sir." Her cheek is on the desk now, her tears running down to puddle on its surface, but her back is arched, presenting her reddened ass for further punishment.

Again. "Ten, sir." She stops sobbing. She's starting to accept her fate, and her stance has widened unconsciously, presenting her pussy to me. Her crotch is so soaked that strands of her juices are dripping down through her underwear.

Again. "Eleven, sir." Her voice has a calmness to it now. She's mine, all mine, and my cock twitches as I envision claiming her.

I raise the belt as high as I can and hold it there a minute as she waits for it, then bring it down full strength. She moans, almost orgasmically. "Twelve, sir."

Dominating a woman is all about being in control, about being calm in the face of intensity, of whatever kind. The calm, in-control thing to do right now is to go down and pay the cabbie for his waiting time while she waits for me in this position, absorbing the lesson I've just inscribed on her ass, on her soul. I already know that I'm going to have her, not just tonight but over and over again, for months, for years, forever. There's no need to hurry into the direct conquest of her body. I know the signs, I can see the relaxation in her face. She'll wait here for me, for as long as I want her to.

But while I am calm, I am not in control, and my cock is painfully erect, and it has been a long time, far too long, since I've had a woman like this. Since before Emily in fact, since that wasn't our relationship. I pull her up, push her down to her knees. She's knows what I want, and her lips are nuzzling my fly immediately. I pull her back by her hair, hard, and she looks up, looking slightly hurt, slightly puzzled...

"Don't you want..."

"Shhhhh..." I put my other forefinger to my lips, holding tight to her hair. "Wait for it."

With deliberate slowness I unzip my fly to free my swelling cock. Her eyes go to it, lock on to it and her desire is clear. Reflexively her lips twitch, parting, and she licks them. She wants it. That's good, I want her to want it. I take it in one hand and tease her with it, running it around her mouth, leaving a glistening strand of seminal fluid to drip from her lower lip. She closes her eyes, inhaling deeply, in rapture. She pulls against the hand holding her hair, but not too hard. She's experiencing her new captivity, exploring the feeling of restraint. She's reliving in her mind all that she's read in my book and her face says it all. She's so ready.

"Mouth open, honey."

She complies, holding her lips wide, forming them into a perfect, inviting O of sexual acceptance. I slide my cock into her, reveling in the warm wetness of her tongue. She closes her lips around me and begins to suck, but I tug harshly on her hair to stop her.

"Just hold it open, honey. Don't suck."

Again she complies, and I see the sudden eroticism of the moment transform her face. She's completely passive now, a pliant sex toy, uninvolved with giving pleasure, simply being used to provide it. Her breathing quickens, and I can see the pulse pounding fast in her throat.

"Tongue out, honey."

She extends her tongue obediently, points it delicately at the head of my cock as I jerk it back and forth. The head rubs against her tongue, taut to the bursting point. There is a point where my cock gets so hard it seems to lose all sensation, as though it were made of steel and not of flesh. It's that hard now, and yet the wet rhythm of her tongue still penetrates to the base of my brain, forcing me to thrust my hips forward. She looks up with big, innocent eyes, mutely imploring me to finish on her, to validate her submission and her desirability in the same sticky instant, to let her know her sacrifice has been rewarded.

I grab her hair again and force my cock deep into her mouth. It is a bestial act, primal, an act of sexual conquest that has no place in a civilized society. I have no illusion that every woman, or even most women, would like the way I am in bed. I have no desire to alter that. I don't want every woman, or even most women. I want this woman, and I want nothing else.

The Writer

The important thing is that she likes it. This interaction is working for her at least as well as it is for me, her nipples are rigidly stiff and the warm, rich scent of feminine musk fills the air.

"Suck it now, honey."

She obliges, and I feel my balls start to contract as I get ready to spill myself into her, onto her. I pump in and out of her lips until I'm ready to burst and then I pull out. She immediately returns to mouth open, tongue extended receptivity, and I'm again jerking myself off on her tongue.

"Beg for it."

She looks up and locks her gaze on mine. "Please come. Sir. Please come on my face." Her voice is pleading, eager and her lips are brushing the head of my cock with every word. "Please, I need it so bad. I'm a dirty little cocksucker and I need you to mark me." She pauses to lick my shaft between every sentence. "Please do it. Please make me your slut. Please let me be your whore."

"Come on, honey, convince me."

Her eyes get big, and she runs her tongue up the underside of my cock. She knows how hot she looks, she knows she can get me off like that.

"Please, Sir." Lick.

"Please I'll do anything." Lick.

"You can fuck me." Lick.

"You can take my ass." Lick.

"You can have me whenever you want." Lick.

"I'll be so good for you." Lick.

"And if I'm not good enough you can punish me." Lick.

"I need it so bad, Sir."

Lick. "*Please!*"

The last *please* is more a groan, half desire and half frustration, and it's all I need to hear. I come, bucking my hips forward to cut off her next sentence as I shoot my juice into her mouth. Like a good girl she doesn't suck, because she hasn't been told to. She just cups her tongue to catch my sperm as I pump in and out of her mouth, my balls contracting so hard they hurt. The waves of pleasure make it impossible to stand and my knees buckle. My cock comes out of her mouth to jet its last spurts on her face, on her lips, and I sink back into her desk chair. She stays kneeling, my sperm on her outstretched tongue, waiting for permission to swallow. She learns fast, this one.

"You can swallow," I tell her, and she does, clearly savouring the taste and texture. Her hair and clothing are in disarray, her face is stained with tears and sperm. What's left on her face drips down over her blouse. She looks the part of the dirty little tramp. She should. She played it well.

I lie back, make an inviting gesture, and she moves over to rest her head in my lap. I stroke her hair affectionately, massage my juices into her skin. She looks up at me with the same big eyes as before. Her face is completely relaxed, as though it were her who had just come through a mind shattering orgasm and not me. I am overwhelmed with emotion, the violent passion of seconds ago replaced with tenderness and concern. I recover my breath enough to speak, let my heart rate slow, and contemplate her beauty for a little while. Eventually I ask the question.

"Would you like me to stay?"

She laughs. "Of course I would. I don't want you to go." She hugs my legs. "Ever."

There's weight in that word. *Ever.* It's far too soon for words like that, so she says it lightly, playfully. At the same time, we both understand the connection here. This is a beginning. I give her the cab fare, and a generous tip, send her down to pay the cabbie. She blushes at the instruction, knowing the cabbie will know from her appearance exactly what has happened. I appreciate her ass as she goes out. While she's gone I move to the couch, take out my laptop and open it, and start to write. The words spill out in an effortless torrent, the story perfect line by line. She comes back, sees me typing and comes to lie down beside me. I move the laptop so she can rest her head on my thigh, watching as my fingers fly over the keys. No words are spoken but we both know the truth. Tonight she has become my muse.

Au Revoir

So you're mine now, honey. You're my very own personal slut, my well trained sex bitch, and I'm going to put you through your paces now. Are you ready? It doesn't matter. Do you remember your lessons? Have you been practicing? I certainly hope so.
Strip.

Au Revoir

Rest.

Au Revoir

Attention:

Au Revoir

Kneel.

Au Revoir

Present.

Au Revoir

Open.

Au Revoir

See how easy it is. Five words and you're on your knees ready to be fucked. Five words and you're ready to take my cock just the way I want you to. You picked this book up with no idea where it would take you, but here you are, through the door and down the road, face down and cunt up. You're mine now, punished and rewarded, trained and restrained. You're my easy, eager, hot little cunt, with your ass in the air whenever I want you, ready to be fucked in any hole, ready to be used, abused, taken, possessed.

Yeah, you do it for me, face down, ass up, that's the way we like to fuck. So do it, fucking do it. Get right down with these words on the floor and your nose on these words. All the way down. Yeah, I love the way I can put you on the floor to be fucked like this. You're already wet. You're that fast, that easy for me. Fuck, I love that.

And now you're going to crawl for me. Don't think, just do it, fucking do it. Keep the book on the floor and your nose on the book and crawl. Keep your knees apart, keep your ass up, and yeah, I want your tits touching the ground. Not easy, is it? Keep crawling, I don't care that it's not easy. I want it to be hard. I want you to feel the effort, I want you to *make* the effort. And you're doing it, because you get it, you understand what I want of you, you understand that you're getting what you need from me. Because no, honey, you don't want it easy from me, do you? No, not at all. Legs wider, bitch. Get your cunt open. Do you want the belt? Maybe not, but you need it. You need it hard. You need your ass welted and your cunt whipped. You need to be put in your place, and this is your place. Face down, cunt up, ready to be impaled on my cock.

Yeah honey, that's the reason you like me so much, that's the reason you love me, because I'm not afraid to give you what you need, even when you're afraid to get it. Yeah I want you. Remember our very first words, way back when the journey began? *Yeah, I want you, spread on my bed like a banquet to feed the hunger of my lust and quench the thirst of my desire.* I want you because fill me, you fulfill me. I want you because you're the most desirable woman I can imagine. I want you because you've passed every one of the tests I've thrown at you, and you're still ready, still eager, still desperate for more. Yeah, I want you, and oh yes, honey, I'm going to have you right now, just take you, just make you do exactly everything you want so much for me to make you do.

You know what to say.
"Yes, sir."
Out loud.
"Yes sir, you can have me, any time, any place, any way, and every way."
Like you mean it.
"Yes sir, you can take me, and I will take it, take it all, take everything."
Convince me.
"Yes sir, I'm yours, I'm all yours and only yours."

Yes, honey. Your body responds to those words, your body responds to me. Your pulse is speeding up, and you can feel your body start to tense. You can feel me here with you, watching you, so close you can almost reach out and touch me. Your lips are begging to be kissed, aching for it. Your skin is getting sensitized, begging to be touched, anywhere and everywhere. You need my hands on you, you need your hands on me. Breathe deep, honey. Breathe deep and inhale my scent, rich and powerful. Your tongue is longing to taste me, to explore my skin. You can feel your breasts swelling in anticipation, there beneath you, pressed against the floor. You can feel your cunt getting wet as your clit stiffens, held up high and presented for whatever I want. Your body knows what it needs, honey, and what it needs is me. You need me on top of you and in between your long, hot legs. You need me inside you, deep, deep inside.

Yeah, you want me. Think about your cervix, honey, that secret spot, the gateway to your womb, the most feminine part of your anatomy. Concentrate on it, feel it throbbing, deep inside. Your cervix has a mission, honey, and that's to kiss the head of my cock, kiss it long and deep and hard. Your cunt longs to be stretched around my cock, forced open and fucked the way it was meant to be fucked. We don't need anything complex here, honey. We don't need the rope, the belt, the riding crop. We don't need the erotic amplification of anal sex or oral sex or lingerie or leather. This is an old, old recipe, shake and bake simple, honey. Add cream to eggs and heat to boiling, stir with a steady, pumping motion, serves two. You're my appetizer and my main course and you're my rich and creamy, hot and steamy, sinfully decadent dream dessert. Cock rigid, cunt wet, in and out and in and out and in and out.

Say it honey. "Please, sir, fuck me hard."

"Please sir, fuck me deep."

"Please sir, fuck me like a bad girl, like a good girl, like a woman, like a slut. Please sir, take me, break me, just make me yours."

Yeah, you're mine. You're my everything, honey, and I need to be inside you so much right now it hurts. I long to consume you, ignite you, immolate you. I want to die screaming in the fire of your passion, I want to have you surround me, surround my cock with your cunt and wrap your long, lean legs around my hips and your arms around my back and pull me into you, just drown me in the whirlpool of your pussy. I want your full, ripe tits in my hands as I drive my cock into you over and over and over. I want you to take it for me honey, I want you to be there, spread and wet and open and I want you to beg with your beautiful lips for me to do it harder, do it faster, do it deeper.

Say it honey. "Harder, faster, deeper."

Say it honey. "Take me, make me, fuck me, fill me."

See it in my eyes, honey, see the need there. Look to the door, the door I could come in through any second. See me there in your mind, see my desire in my eyes and the huge bulge in my pants. Four quick strides to get to you, to push you down and mount you, to tear my way through whatever is in my way and then, oh yes, and then my rigid cock comes free, your ass coming up and open and that first beautiful touch of cock and cunt, pushing into your wetness, claiming your most intimate territory, while you gasp and groan and push your hips back to open yourself more, to get it deeper inside you. Feel your womb contract and throb at that penetration, that violation, that consummation. Feel your nipples swell and harden, feel your clit explode. And I care about none of that, honey, because my whole world, my universe is your cunt.

Fuck yes, honey. Deep, deep inside. Feel your hips start to move in response, feel yourself open up for me, feel your clit get harder still. Yeah, you can rub it, honey. You can stroke it, because I love the way you wiggle when you do. I love the way you gasp and sigh and the way the pleasure zips through your body. I love the way you get wet and wetter, sluttier, dirtier. I love the way your voice drops, I love the way it tenses up.

"Please, please fuck me." Say it honey.

"Please, please fuck me hard and deep and fast."

And yes, honey, yes I will. My balls are swelling, heavy laden with your special present, ready to be injected right into your very center, right into your core.

"Please, please fuck me."

"Please, please come inside me, right inside me, deep inside me."

"Please, please fuck me, fill me, finish me."

Yeah, honey, what I need right now is you and any second you're going to get it, get that lake of hot white sperm flooding in and up and over. That's the image that's driving me now, forcing the blood down into my cock, making it steel hard and fucking huge. That's the image that's forcing me to fuck it into you, over and over and over. I love the smack of my pelvis on your ass, the feel of your stiffly presented clit against me there. It's wild and raw, honey. It's what has to happen, the logical conclusion and there is nothing in this world that's going to stop me now. Nothing. I'm going to ride you hard and put you away wet. Very, very, wet.

Yeah, honey, you're so feminine at that moment, that ultimate moment when I unload into you. You're so fucking hot, the quintessential woman, slut, bitch, queen, witch, you're everything. And there's just one thing I need in this world right now, one thing I need to finish inside you, pump my balls into your willing open cunt until, and that is to see you come beneath me, feel you give it all up, hear you fucking scream for me. So do it, fucking do it. Do it for me, honey. Do it hard and deep and fast, fucking come for me. Do it, fucking do it.

Do it right. Do it right now.

Now!

Au Revoir

And do you know what I love more than anything, honey? I love that long, long moment after I've spent myself inside you, that long, long moment while you're still shuddering through your own climax, crying out, crying, overwhelmed by the experience. I love being inside you then, staying inside you, feeling your body tense and release, tense and release. Fuck, that's beautiful, fuck, you're beautiful. And all I want at this moment is your skin next to me, to kiss you, to hold you, to reach down and feel where we're still connected by my erection. I want you to breathe deep and come down with me, stay awhile in this little secret spot we share. We have so little time together, honey. Every moment is precious. Let me hold you, honey, let me keep you close and safe.

In a while time will catch up to us, in a while life will call you away. You're going to read my words again, I know that much. You're going to read them over and over and over, but you can never again read them for the first time. This has been our first time, honey, and I know you think it's over now, because this is the end of the book, end of the journey. *Au revoir* is what the French say for *Goodbye,* but that isn't what it means. You've come through the door, you're in the middle of our road, but like Bambi in the headlights, you don't know that it's too late to dodge the truck. You're sitting there all warm and post-orgasmic, and you think this is only not-quite-so-innocent masturbation, private sex, us alone in our separate times, separate spaces, alone with our fantasies. You think these are only words, but honey, words have power, words change lives, and my words have just changed your life you have only two choices.

You aren't reading this when and where I'm writing it, but I'm just as real as you are, honey. I'm flesh and blood, muscle and bone, tall and dark and lean. I'm everything you can imagine and I'm a whole lot more you can't. And I am out here, right here, right now. You know me now honey, and because you're still reading I know you. I know how different you are from the women who've put this book down, the women who never picked it up. I know your secrets and your passions and your dreams, and most of all I know that you're mine. You're fascinated by our little interaction, compelled by it, and you want *more*, you need *more*, and now you know that *more* is right here, right now, waiting just for you.

You see, honey, *Au revoir* means *until I see you again.* Our journey isn't ending now, it's only just begun. So choice one is to do exactly what you're thinking right now, which is apply your mind, and your determination, and find out exactly who it is standing behind these words, who it is who can seize your mind, who it is who can compel your body, who it is who can possess your soul before we've even met. And choice two is - just walk away. Just walk away and wonder forever what would have happened if you'd chosen option one. And either way I have gotten exactly what I want from you because the kind of woman I need is exactly the kind of woman with the brains to figure out the challenge, the confidence to handle it, and the determination to make it happen.

You have the tools, honey, you have that letter you've written me, those photos you took, the homework you did. You've passed every test but the last one, and now I have just one question left. Are you *her*, honey? You already know the answer, deep, deep inside your mind, and no matter what it is, that answer is about to change your life. So if you're not her, I hope it's been as good for you to read this as it has been for me to write it, and that's very, very good indeed. And if you are her, well, the door is open, the road is in front of you. Who knows where it might lead?

Au revoir.

END